SUPER EASY DIABETIC DIET COOKBOOK AFTER 50

Nutritious And Healthy Low-Sugar, Low-Carb And High-Fiber Recipes for Seniors with Pre-Diabetes and Type 2 Diabetes

Kimberly Mullins

I just wanted to drop you a quick note to say a huge thank you for buying my book. Your support really means a lot to me, and I hope you find the recipes helpful and enjoyable.

DISCLAIMER

The information provided in this communication is for general information only. It should not be considered as professional, legal, medical, or financial advice. You are encouraged to seek advice and confirmation from qualified experts or professionals before making any decisions or taking actions based on the content provided here. We do not guarantee the accuracy, completeness, or suitability of the information and shall not be liable for any errors, omissions, or damages arising from its use. Any reliance you place on this information is strictly at your own risk. This communication does not create a professional-client relationship. Any views or opinions expressed here are solely those of the individual author and do not necessarily represent the views of any organization or entity. We reserve the right to modify, update, or remove content at any time without notice. By continuing to read or interact with this content, you agree to these terms and conditions.

ABOUT THE AUTHOR

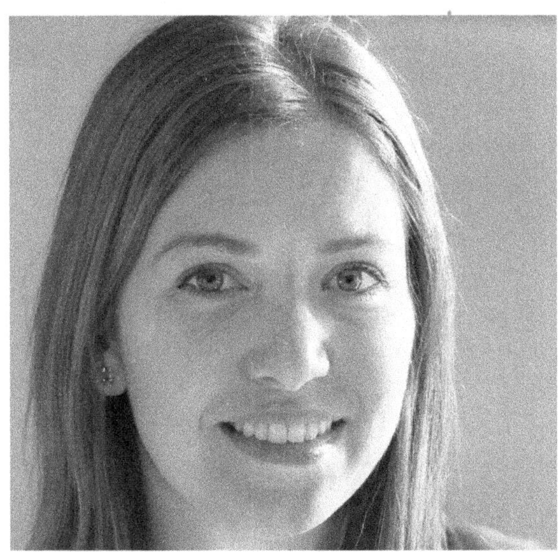

Kimberly Mullins is a renowned chef and dedicated dietitian with a passion for promoting healthy eating and lifestyle choices. With a culinary flair and a deep understanding of nutrition, she has made it her mission to inspire individuals and families to lead happier, healthier lives through the food they consume.

As a chef, Kimberly's expertise lies in crafting delectable dishes that not only tantalize the taste buds but also nourish the body. Her culinary creations seamlessly blend flavors, textures, and ingredients to make wholesome meals that cater to a wide range of dietary preferences and restrictions.

Simultaneously, Kimberly's background as a dietitian empowers her to provide sound nutritional advice and guidance. She understands the intricate relationship between food and well-being and strives to educate others on making informed choices for optimal health.

Beyond her professional pursuits, Kimberly is a loving wife and a devoted mother of two. Her own family serves as the cornerstone of her commitment to health and wellness, driving her to explore creative ways to make nutritious eating an enjoyable and integral part of daily life.

Kimberly Mullins' journey in the culinary and dietary world has led her to become a trusted source of expertise, helping countless individuals and families embrace a lifestyle that prioritizes health, balance, and deliciousness. Through her writing and culinary creations, she continues to inspire and guide others toward a more vibrant and wholesome way of living

DEDICATION

To all those who have gracefully embraced the golden years and are determined to live them to the fullest. May this book be a beacon of hope and a guide to a healthier, sweeter life without the sugar. Your strength and resilience are the true inspirations behind these pages. Let this be your companion on the journey to well-being, for it is never too late to prioritize your health and savor every moment with vitality and joy.

TABLE OF CONTENTS

INTRODUCTION

Life is a journey filled with twists and turns, and as we celebrate the milestone of reaching 50 and beyond, our focus naturally shifts towards nurturing our well-being. It's a time to reflect on our health journey and embrace the wisdom that comes with age. For many of us, managing diabetes becomes an important part of this journey—a challenge that requires thoughtful attention and adaptation.

I'm Kimberly Mullins, a passionate dietitian dedicated to helping individuals live healthier lives through delicious and nutritious food choices. In this cookbook, I invite you to join me on a flavorful exploration of diabetic-friendly eating tailored specifically for those over 50.

The recipes you'll discover here are more than just meals—they're expressions of joy, flavor, and nourishment. From energizing breakfasts to comforting dinners and delightful desserts, each dish is crafted with your health and taste buds in mind.

But this cookbook is about more than recipes; it's a guide to thriving with diabetes after 50. Throughout these pages.

<u>Understanding Diabetes after 50</u>

As we reach the age of 50 and beyond, our bodies undergo natural changes that can impact our health and well-being, including an increased risk of developing certain health conditions such as diabetes. Diabetes is a complex metabolic disorder characterized by high blood sugar levels, and its management requires a nuanced understanding, especially in the context of aging.

One of the key considerations in understanding diabetes after 50 is recognizing the role of lifestyle factors and genetic predisposition. As we age, our bodies may become less efficient in processing sugars, which can contribute to insulin resistance or reduced insulin production, leading to diabetes. Additionally, factors such as sedentary lifestyle, poor dietary choices over the years, and changes in hormone levels can further influence diabetes risk.

It's important to acknowledge that managing diabetes after 50 requires a holistic approach that goes beyond blood sugar control. This includes addressing other health concerns that commonly coexist with diabetes in older adults, such as high blood pressure, cholesterol imbalances, and cardiovascular complications.

Emotionally, a diabetes diagnosis after 50 can be daunting. It may bring about feelings of uncertainty, fear, or frustration. However, it's crucial to recognize that diabetes is a manageable condition with the right knowledge, support, and lifestyle modifications.

For individuals over 50, understanding diabetes involves learning about the importance of balanced nutrition, regular physical activity, stress management, and medication adherence. It's about empowering oneself with knowledge and adopting practical strategies to live well with diabetes.

Importance of Diet and Lifestyle in Managing Diabetes

Managing diabetes is not just about monitoring blood sugar levels or taking medications—it's about embracing a holistic approach to health that encompasses both diet and lifestyle choices. For individuals with diabetes, particularly those over the age of 50, the significance of diet and lifestyle cannot be overstated.

Diet plays a central role in diabetes management, influencing blood sugar levels, insulin sensitivity, and overall health outcomes. By making informed food choices and adopting a balanced eating pattern, individuals with diabetes can better control their blood sugar levels and reduce the risk of complications.

But what does a diabetes-friendly diet look like? It's about focusing on whole, nutrient-rich foods while minimizing processed foods, sugary beverages, and refined carbohydrates. Emphasizing fiber-rich fruits and vegetables, lean proteins, whole grains, and healthy fats can help stabilize blood sugar levels and promote overall well-being.

Yet, the importance of lifestyle factors extends beyond diet alone. Regular physical activity is another cornerstone of diabetes management, offering a myriad of benefits such as improved insulin sensitivity, weight management, and cardiovascular health. Engaging in regular exercise not only helps control blood sugar levels but also boosts mood, energy levels, and overall quality of life.

Furthermore, managing stress, getting adequate sleep, and maintaining a healthy weight are all integral components of a comprehensive diabetes management plan. Chronic stress and poor sleep quality can negatively impact blood sugar control and contribute to insulin resistance, while excess weight can increase the risk of complications associated with diabetes.

Emotionally, embracing diet and lifestyle changes to manage diabetes can be challenging. It may require adjusting long-standing habits, navigating social situations, and overcoming barriers to change. However, it's important to approach this journey with compassion, patience, and a commitment to self-care.

CHAPTER 1: NUTRITIONAL GUIDELINES FOR DIABETES MANAGEMENT

Importance of Balanced Nutrition

Balanced nutrition plays a crucial role in managing diabetes and promoting overall health and well-being. Here are some key reasons why balanced nutrition is important:

1. Blood Sugar Control: Consuming a balanced diet that includes a variety of nutrient-rich foods helps regulate blood sugar levels and prevents spikes and crashes. Balancing carbohydrates, proteins, and fats in each meal can help stabilize blood sugar levels and reduce the risk of hyperglycemia (high blood sugar) and hypoglycemia (low blood sugar).

2. Weight Management: A balanced diet supports weight management efforts, which is important for individuals with diabetes, particularly those who are overweight or obese. Maintaining a healthy weight can improve insulin sensitivity, reduce the risk of insulin resistance, and lower the likelihood of complications associated with diabetes, such as cardiovascular disease and neuropathy.

3. Nutrient Intake: Consuming a variety of nutrient-rich foods ensures that individuals with diabetes receive essential vitamins, minerals, antioxidants, and phytonutrients necessary for optimal health and functioning. Fruits, vegetables, whole grains, lean proteins, and healthy fats provide essential nutrients that support immune function, tissue repair, and overall vitality.

4. Heart Health: A balanced diet that emphasizes whole foods, fiber-rich plant foods, and healthy fats supports heart health and reduces the risk of cardiovascular complications associated with diabetes. Consuming foods rich in omega-3 fatty acids, such as fatty fish, nuts, and seeds, can help lower triglyceride levels, reduce inflammation, and improve lipid profiles.

5. Gut Health: The gut microbiome plays a key role in regulating metabolism, immune function, and inflammation, all of which are relevant to diabetes management. Consuming a balanced diet that includes prebiotic-rich foods (such as fruits, vegetables, and whole grains) and probiotic-containing foods (such as yogurt and fermented foods) promotes a healthy gut microbiome and may improve glucose metabolism.

6. Energy and Vitality: Balanced nutrition provides the energy and nutrients needed for optimal physical and cognitive function, supporting overall energy levels, mental clarity, and vitality. Maintaining stable blood sugar levels through balanced meals and snacks can help prevent fatigue, mood swings, and cognitive decline associated with blood sugar fluctuations.

7. Long-Term Health: Adopting a balanced diet as part of a healthy lifestyle promotes long-term health and reduces the risk of chronic diseases beyond diabetes, such as cancer, osteoporosis, and age-related cognitive decline. Eating a variety of nutrient-dense foods and minimizing processed foods, added sugars, and unhealthy fats supports overall well-being and longevity.

The Role of Protein, Fat, and Fiber in Diabetes Management

I often emphasize the importance of understanding the role that different nutrients play in supporting blood sugar control and overall well-being. Protein, fat, and fiber are three key nutrients that can have a profound impact on managing diabetes and promoting optimal health.

• **Protein:** Protein is necessary for immune system support, tissue growth and repair and muscle mass maintenance. For individuals with diabetes, incorporating adequate protein into meals and snacks can help stabilize blood sugar levels, promote satiety, and prevent spikes in insulin secretion.

But the role of protein extends beyond blood sugar control. It can also play a crucial role in weight management, as protein-rich foods tend to be more filling and satisfying than carbohydrates or fats. This can help individuals with diabetes manage their appetite, reduce cravings for unhealthy foods, and support weight loss or weight maintenance goals.

However, it's important to choose lean sources of protein, such as poultry, fish, lean cuts of meat, tofu, tempeh, legumes, and low-fat dairy products, to minimize saturated fat intake and promote heart health.

• **<u>Fat</u>:** Fat is another important nutrient that plays a significant role in diabetes management. While it's often vilified, especially in the context of heart health, not all fats are created equal. Healthy fats, such as monounsaturated and polyunsaturated fats found in nuts, seeds, avocados, and olive oil, can have beneficial effects on blood sugar control, insulin sensitivity, and cardiovascular health.

Incorporating healthy fats into meals can help slow down the absorption of carbohydrates, leading to more gradual increases in blood sugar levels and improved glycemic control. Additionally, fat-rich foods can contribute to feelings of satiety and satisfaction, which can help individuals with diabetes manage their appetite and food intake.

• **Fiber:** Plant-based foods contain a kind of carbohydrate called fiber, which the body is unable to completely digest. It plays a crucial role in regulating blood sugar levels, promoting digestive health, and supporting weight management. Fiber-rich foods, such as fruits, vegetables, whole grains, legumes, nuts, and seeds, help slow down the absorption of glucose into the bloodstream, leading to more stable blood sugar levels after meals.

In addition to its blood sugar-lowering effects, fiber adds bulk to the diet, promoting feelings of fullness and reducing overall calorie intake. This can be particularly beneficial for individuals with diabetes who are trying to lose weight or control their appetite.

Foods to Eat

1. Non-Starchy Vegetables: Fill half your plate with non-starchy vegetables such as leafy greens, broccoli, cauliflower, bell peppers, cucumbers, and tomatoes. These foods are low in carbohydrates and calories, rich in fiber, vitamins, and minerals, and help promote satiety.

2. Whole Grains: Choose whole grains such as quinoa, brown rice, barley, oats, and whole wheat bread and pasta. Whole grains are rich in fiber, which slows down the absorption of carbohydrates and helps stabilize blood sugar levels.

3. Lean Proteins: Include lean protein sources in your meals, such as skinless poultry, fish, tofu, tempeh, legumes, and low-fat dairy products. Protein helps promote satiety, supports muscle health, and does not significantly impact blood sugar levels.

4. Healthy Fats: Incorporate sources of healthy fats into your diet, such as avocados, nuts, seeds, olive oil, and fatty fish like salmon and mackerel. Healthy fats help improve insulin sensitivity, promote heart health, and provide essential nutrients.

5. Low-Fat Dairy: Choose low-fat or fat-free dairy products such as skim milk, yogurt, and cheese. Dairy products provide essential nutrients like calcium and vitamin D while keeping saturated fat intake in check.

6. Herbs and Spices: Flavor your meals with herbs, spices, and seasonings instead of salt and sugar. Herbs and spices add depth and flavor to dishes without adding extra calories or carbohydrates.

Foods to Limit

1. Processed Foods: Limit processed foods such as packaged snacks, sugary cereals, processed meats, and convenience meals. These foods are often high in added sugars, unhealthy fats, and sodium, which can negatively impact blood sugar control and overall health.

2. Sugary Beverages: Limit or avoid sugary beverages such as soda, fruit juices, sweetened teas, and energy drinks. These drinks include a lot of added sugar and can quickly raise blood sugar levels.

3. Sweets and Desserts: Limit sweets and desserts such as cakes, cookies, pastries, and ice cream to occasional treats. These foods are high in sugar and refined carbohydrates, which can lead to blood sugar spikes and contribute to weight gain if consumed in excess.

4. High-Sodium Foods: Limit foods high in sodium, such as canned soups, salty snacks, processed meats, and fast food. High sodium intake can increase the risk of high blood pressure and cardiovascular complications, especially for individuals with diabetes.

Foods to Avoid

1. Trans Fats: Avoid foods high in trans fats, such as fried foods, packaged snacks, and baked goods made with partially hydrogenated oils. Trans fats raise LDL (bad) cholesterol levels and increase the risk of heart disease and stroke.

2. Excessive Alcohol: Limit alcohol consumption to moderate amounts, if at all. Excessive alcohol intake can interfere with blood sugar control, increase the risk of hypoglycemia, and contribute to weight gain.

3. High-Glycemic Foods: Limit high-glycemic foods such as white bread, white rice, sugary cereals, and refined grains. These foods can cause rapid spikes in blood sugar levels and should be consumed in moderation.

Fruits to Eat

• **Berries (e.g., strawberries, blueberries, raspberries):** Berries are rich in antioxidants, fiber, and vitamins while having a relatively low impact on blood sugar levels.

• **Cherries:** Cherries are low in calories and have a moderate glycemic index, making them a good choice for individuals with diabetes.
• **Apples:** Apples are high in fiber, which can help slow down the absorption of sugar into the bloodstream.
• **Pears:** Pears are another good source of fiber and have a lower glycemic index compared to some other fruits.
• **Citrus fruits (e.g., oranges, grapefruits, lemons, limes):** Citrus fruits are rich in vitamin C and fiber and tend to have a lower glycemic index.

Fruits to Consume in Moderation

• **Bananas:** While bananas are nutritious and provide potassium, they are higher in carbohydrates and can cause a more significant rise in blood sugar levels.
• **Grapes**: Grapes are convenient and tasty but are relatively high in natural sugars. Limit portion sizes to manage blood sugar levels.
• **Mangoes**: Mangoes are delicious but can be higher in sugar compared to other fruits. Enjoy in moderation and consider pairing with protein or healthy fats to slow sugar absorption.

Fruits to Avoid or Limit

• **Dried fruits (e.g., raisins, dates, dried apricots):** Dried fruits are concentrated sources of sugar and can cause rapid spikes in blood sugar levels. Choose fresh fruits instead.
- **Pineapple:** Pineapple is relatively high in natural sugars and has a moderate to high glycemic index.
• **Watermelon:** Watermelon is high in natural sugars and has a high glycemic index. Enjoy in small portions and pair with protein or healthy fats.
• **Fruit juices:** Fruit juices can cause rapid spikes in blood sugar levels due to their high sugar content. Opt for whole fruits instead.

CHAPTER 2: QUICK BREAKFAST RECIPES

Coconut Muffins

Prep Time: 10 minutes

Cook Time: 20 minutes

Servings: 12 muffins

Ingredients
- 1 cup whole wheat flour
- 1/2 cup almond flour
- 1/4 cup coconut flour
- 1/2 cup unsweetened shredded coconut
- 1 teaspoon baking powder
- 1/2 teaspoon baking soda
- 1/4 teaspoon salt
- 2 large eggs
- 1/4 cup honey or maple syrup (for sweetness)
- 1/4 cup coconut oil, melted
- One cup of unsweetened coconut milk or almond milk
- 1 teaspoon vanilla extract

Instructions

1. Set a muffin tray with paper liners or lightly spray with coconut oil and preheat the oven to 350°F (175°C).

2. Place the whole wheat flour, almond flour, coconut flour, shredded coconut, baking soda, baking powder, and salt in a large mixing bowl. Mix thoroughly until fully incorporated.

3. In another dish, mix together the eggs, melted coconut oil, coconut milk, vanilla extract, honey or maple syrup, until smooth.

4. Add the liquid mixture to the dry mixture and gently fold just until incorporated. Be careful not to blend too much.

5. Evenly distribute the batter into each muffin cup, filling it to about two thirds of the way.

6. Bake for 18 to 20 minutes in a preheated oven, or until a toothpick inserted into the muffins comes out clean.

7. Remove from the oven and allow the muffins to cool in the pan for a few minutes before transferring them to a wire rack to cool completely.

Nutritional Information (per muffin):
- Calories: 180
- Total Fat: 10g
- Saturated Fat: 7g
- Cholesterol: 35mg
- Sodium: 110mg
- Total Carbohydrates: 19g
- Dietary Fiber: 3g
- Sugars: 7g
- Protein: 4g

Ingredient Substitutions
- For a gluten-free option, replace the whole wheat flour with gluten-free flour blend or oat flour.
- Swap almond flour with more whole wheat flour or oat flour if desired.
- Use agave nectar or stevia as a sugar substitute for a lower glycemic index.

Almond Flour Banana Bread

Prep Time: 15 minutes

Cook Time: 50 minutes

- Servings: 10 slices

Ingredients:
- 2 ripe bananas, mashed
- 3 large eggs
- 1/4 cup coconut oil, melted
- 1/4 cup honey or maple syrup
- 1 teaspoon vanilla extract
- 2 cups almond flour
- 1 teaspoon baking powder
- 1/2 teaspoon baking soda
- 1/4 teaspoon salt
- Sprinkles (optional, for garnish)

Instructions:

1. Preheat your oven to 350°F (175°C) and grease a 9x5-inch loaf pan with coconut oil or line it with parchment paper.

2. In a large mixing bowl, combine the mashed bananas, eggs, melted coconut oil, honey or maple syrup, and vanilla extract. Whisk until well combined.

3. In another dish mix together the almond flour, baking powder, baking soda, and salt.

4. Add the liquid mixture to the dry mixture and gently fold just until incorporated. Take caution not to blend too much.

5. Pour the batter into the prepared loaf pan, spreading it out evenly.

6. If desired, sprinkle the top of the batter with colorful sprinkles for a festive touch.

7. Bake for 45-50 minutes in a preheated oven, or until a toothpick inserted into the muffins comes out clean.

8. Remove from the oven and allow the banana bread to cool in the pan for 10-15 minutes before transferring it to a wire rack to cool completely.

Nutritional Information (per slice):
- Calories: 200
- Total Fat: 15g
- Saturated Fat: 5g
- Cholesterol: 50mg
- Sodium: 150mg
- Total Carbohydrates: 15g
- Dietary Fiber: 3g
- Sugars: 8g
- Protein: 6g

Ingredient Substitutions:
- For a vegan option, replace the eggs with flax eggs (1 tablespoon ground flaxseed meal + 3 tablespoons water per egg).
- Use melted butter or avocado oil instead of coconut oil if preferred.
- Substitute maple syrup with agave nectar or date syrup for a vegan alternative.

Curry-Avocado Crispy Egg Toast

Prep Time: 10 minutes
Cook Time: 5 minutes
Servings: 2 toasts

Ingredients:

- 2 slices whole grain bread
- 1 ripe avocado, mashed
- 2 large eggs
- 1 teaspoon curry powder
- 1/4 teaspoon garlic powder
- 1/4 teaspoon onion powder
- Salt and pepper, to taste
- Cooking spray or olive oil

Instructions:

1. A non-stick skillet should be heated to medium heat and lightly oiled or coated with cooking spray.

2. Combine the eggs, curry powder, onion powder, garlic powder, salt, and pepper in a small bowl and whisk until thoroughly mixed.

3. Transfer the egg mixture onto the skillet and level it out so that a thin layer forms.

4. Cook the eggs for two to three minutes, or until the bottoms are set and have a hint of color.

5. Cook the eggs for a further one to two minutes, or until they are thoroughly cooked, after carefully flipping them. Take out and place aside from the skillet.

6. Toast the whole grain bread slices until crispy and golden brown.

7. Evenly distribute the mashed avocado over each piece of toast.

8. Transfer the fried eggs with curry powder on top of the mashed avocado

9. Garnish with additional salt, pepper, and a sprinkle of curry powder if desired.

Nutritional Information (per serving):
- Calories: 320
- Total Fat: 18g

- Saturated Fat: 3.5g
- Cholesterol: 185mg
- Sodium: 320mg
- Total Carbohydrates: 29g
- Dietary Fiber: 9g
- Sugars: 3g
- Protein: 15g

Ingredient Substitutions:
- Use gluten-free bread for a gluten-free option.
- Customize the level of spice by adjusting the amount of curry powder to suit your taste preferences.
- Add sliced tomatoes or greens such as spinach or arugula for extra freshness and nutrients.

Oatmeal Pancakes with Maple Fruit

Prep Time: 15 minutes

Cook Time: 15 minutes

Servings: 4 pancakes

Ingredients:
For the Pancakes:
- 1 cup old-fashioned oats
- 1 cup whole wheat flour
- 2 teaspoons baking powder
- 1/2 teaspoon ground cinnamon
- 1/4 teaspoon salt
- 1 ripe banana, mashed
- 1 cup unsweetened almond milk (or any milk of your choice)
- 2 tablespoons maple syrup
- 1 large egg
- 1 teaspoon vanilla extract

- Coconut oil or cooking spray

For the Maple Fruit:
- One cup of mixed berries such as strawberries, blueberries, and raspberries
- 2 tablespoons pure maple syrup
- 1 tablespoon lemon juice
- 1/4 teaspoon vanilla extract

Instructions:
1. To produce oat flour, pulse the oats in a blender or food processor until they are finely pulverized.

2. Combine the oat flour, whole wheat flour, baking powder, cinnamon, and salt in a sizable mixing basin.

3. In another dish, blend the almond milk, egg, maple syrup, mashed banana, and vanilla extract until smooth.

4. Add the liquid mixture to the dry mixture and whisk just until blended. Be careful not to blend too much.

5. Turn up the heat to medium and give a non-stick skillet or griddle a quick coat of cooking spray or coconut oil.

6. For each pancake, add roughly 1/4 cup of batter to the griddle. When bubbles start to form on the surface, turn the food over and cook it until the second side is golden brown.

7. Repeat with the remaining batter, adding more cooking spray or oil to the skillet as needed.

For the Maple Fruit:
1. The mixed berries, maple syrup, lemon juice, and vanilla extract should all be combined in a small pot.
2. Cook for 5 to 7 minutes over medium heat, stirring periodically, or until the berries soften and release their juices.
3. Before serving, remove from the heat and allow it to cool slightly.

Nutritional Information (per serving, including maple fruit):
- Calories: 280
- Total Fat: 3g
- Saturated Fat: 0.5g
- Cholesterol: 35mg
- Sodium: 320mg
- Total Carbohydrates: 56g
- Dietary Fiber: 7g
- Sugars: 18g
- Protein: 9g

Ingredient Substitutions:
- Use gluten-free oats or oat flour for a gluten-free option.
- Substitute mashed sweet potato or applesauce for the mashed banana if desired.
- Swap the almond milk with any milk of your choice, such as dairy milk, soy milk, or oat milk.

Peanut Butter & Berries Waffle Sandwich

Prep Time: 5 minutes
Cook Time: 5 minutes

Servings: 1 sandwich

Ingredients:
- 4 whole grain waffles (homemade or store-bought)
- 1/4 cup natural peanut butter (smooth or crunchy)
- One cup of mixed berries such as strawberries, blueberries, and raspberries
- 1 tablespoon honey or maple syrup (optional, for drizzling)
- Fresh mint leaves, for garnish (optional)

Instructions:

1. Toast the whole grain waffles until golden brown and crispy.

2. Spread a generous layer of peanut butter onto two of the toasted waffles.

3. Top the peanut butter-coated waffles with a handful of mixed berries, spreading them out evenly.

4. Drizzle honey or maple syrup over the berries if desired, for an extra touch of sweetness.

5. Place the remaining two toasted waffles on top of the berry-covered waffles to form sandwiches.

6. Gently press down to secure the sandwiches.

Nutritional Information (per sandwich):
- Calories: 320
- Total Fat: 16g
- Saturated Fat: 3g
- Cholesterol: 0mg
- Sodium: 260mg
- Total Carbohydrates: 38g
- Dietary Fiber: 6g
- Sugars: 12g
- Protein: 10g

Ingredient Substitutions:
- Use gluten-free waffles for a gluten-free option.
- If desired, substitute cashew butter or almond butter for peanut butter
- Swap the mixed berries with sliced bananas or other favorite fruits for variety.

Southwest Breakfast Quesadilla

Prep Time: 10 minutes
Cook Time: 10 minutes
Servings: 1 quesadilla

Ingredients:
- Two big corn tortillas or whole wheat
- 2 large eggs, scrambled
- 1/4 cup black beans, drained and rinsed
- 1/4 cup diced bell peppers (any color)
- 2 tablespoons diced red onion
- 1/4 cup shredded cheddar or Monterey Jack cheese
- 1/2 avocado, sliced
- Salsa, for serving
- Fresh cilantro, for garnish (optional)
- Cooking spray or olive oil

Instructions:
A non-stick skillet should be heated to medium heat and lightly oiled or coated with cooking spray.

2. Put one tortilla in the skillet and equally top it with half of the scrambled eggs.

3. Top the eggs with half of the shredded cheese, diced bell peppers, red onion, and black beans.

4. To close the quesadilla, place the remaining tortilla on top and gently press down with a spatula.

5. Cook the tortilla for two to three minutes on each side, or until the cheese has melted and the tortilla is crispy and golden brown.

6. Take out of the skillet and place the quesadilla on a chopping board.

7. If preferred, garnish the quesadilla with sliced avocado, salsa, and fresh cilantro after slicing it into wedges.

Nutritional Information (per quesadilla):
- Calories: 380
- Total Fat: 20g
- Saturated Fat: 6g
- Cholesterol: 210mg
- Sodium: 430mg
- Total Carbohydrates: 32g
- Dietary Fiber: 9g
- Sugars: 2g
- Protein: 20g

Ingredient Substitutions:
- Use whole grain or gluten-free tortillas for a healthier or gluten-free option.
- Substitute pinto beans or refried beans for black beans if preferred.
- Customize the filing with your favorite vegetables such as spinach, tomatoes, or mushrooms.

Healthy Herb Frittata

Prep Time: 10 minutes
Cook Time: 15 minutes
Servings: 2 servings

Ingredients:
- 6 large eggs
- 1/4 cup milk (dairy or non-dairy)
- 1 cup chopped mixed vegetables (such as bell peppers, onions, spinach, and tomatoes)
- 2 tablespoons chopped fresh herbs (such as parsley, basil, chives, and thyme)

- 1/4 cup shredded cheese (such as cheddar, feta, or goat cheese)
- Salt and pepper, to taste
- Cooking spray or olive oil

Instructions:

1. Set the oven temperature to 350°F (175°C).

2. Beat the eggs and milk together thoroughly in a sizable mixing dish. To taste, add salt and pepper for seasoning.

3. Lightly spray or cover a nonstick skillet with olive oil or cooking spray before heating it over medium heat.

4. Add the chopped mixed vegetables to the skillet and cook for about five minutes, or until they are soft.

5. Ensure that the veggies are equally distributed by pouring the egg mixture over them in the skillet.

6. Evenly distribute the shredded cheese and finely chopped fresh herbs on top of the frittata.

7. On a burner, cook a frittata for three to four minutes, or until the edges start to set.

8. Place the skillet in the oven and bake for ten to twelve minutes, or until the frittata is set in the center and lightly golden brown on top.

9. Take out of the oven and let it cool down a little before slicing it into wedges.

Nutritional Information (per serving):
- Calories: 150
- Total Fat: 10g
- Saturated Fat: 4g
- Cholesterol: 190 mg
- Sodium: 230mg
- Total Carbohydrates: 4g

- Dietary Fiber: 1g
- Sugars: 2g
- Protein: 11g

Ingredient Substitutions:
- Use any combination of your favorite vegetables and herbs for variety.
- Substitute dairy milk with almond milk, coconut milk, or any other non-dairy milk alternative.
- Omit the cheese for a dairy-free option or use a vegan cheese alternative if preferred.

Spinach & Egg Scramble with Raspberries

Prep Time: 5 minutes
Cook Time: 10 minutes
Servings: 1 serving

Ingredients:
- 2 large eggs
- 1 cup fresh baby spinach leaves
- One quarter cup of diced red bell pepper
- 1/4 cup diced red onion
- 1 tablespoon olive oil or cooking spray
- Salt and pepper, to taste
- 1/2 cup fresh raspberries
- Fresh herbs (such as parsley or chives), for garnish (optional)

Instructions:
1. Beat the eggs thoroughly in a small bowl. Add salt and pepper for seasoning.

2. In a nonstick skillet over medium heat, warm up some olive oil or cooking spray.

3. Add the chopped red onion and bell pepper to the skillet and cook for two to three minutes, or until the vegetables are tender.

4. Cook the fresh baby spinach leaves in the skillet for one to two minutes, or until they have wilted.

5. Scramble the veggies in the skillet by pouring the beaten eggs over them and gently stirring.

6. Cook for two to three minutes, or until the eggs are set but still somewhat wet.

7. Take the skillet off of the burner and place the scrambled eggs onto a platter.

8. Place the fresh raspberries next to the eggs that have been scrambled.

9. Accent with fresh herbs, if desired

Nutritional Information (per serving):
- Calories: 210
- Total Fat: 13g
- Saturated Fat: 3g
- Cholesterol: 370mg
- Sodium: 280mg
- Total Carbohydrates: 11g
- Dietary Fiber: 5g
- Sugars: 5g
- Protein: 13g

Ingredient Substitutions:
- Use any leafy greens such as kale or Swiss chard instead of spinach.
- Substitute diced tomatoes or mushrooms for the red bell pepper if preferred.
- Replace raspberries with strawberries, blueberries, or any other favorite fruit for variety.

Pistachio & Peach Toast

Prep Time: 5 minutes

Cook Time: 5 minutes

Servings: 1 toast

Ingredients:
- 1 slice whole grain bread, toasted
- 2 tablespoons pistachio butter (or almond butter)
- 1 ripe peach, thinly sliced
- 1 tablespoon chopped pistachios, for garnish
- Drizzle of honey(optional)

Instructions:

1. Toast the whole grain bread slice till it is crispy and golden brown.

2. Evenly distribute the pistachio butter over the toast.

3. Place the thinly sliced peach over the butter with pistachios.

4. To add more crunchy and taste to the peach slices, sprinkle chopped pistachios on top.

5. If desired, drizzle with honey to add even more sweetness.

Nutritional Information (per serving):
- Calories: 240
- Total Fat: 12g
- Saturated Fat: 1.5g
- Cholesterol: 0mg
- Sodium: 170mg
- Total Carbohydrates: 30g

Savory Oatmeal with Tomato & Sausage

Prep Time: 5 minutes
Cook Time: 10 minutes
Servings: 1 serving

Ingredients:
- 1/2 cup old-fashioned oats
- 1 cup water or low-sodium chicken broth
- One quarter cup of fresh or canned diced tomatoes
- 2 cooked sausage links, sliced (turkey, chicken, or pork)
- 1/4 teaspoon garlic powder
- 1/4 teaspoon dried oregano
- Salt and pepper, to taste
- Fresh basil leaves, for garnish (optional)
- Grated Parmesan cheese, for garnish (optional)

Instructions:
1. Heat the chicken broth or water in a small saucepan until it boils.

2. Turn down the heat and stir in the oats. Cook for 5 to 7 minutes, stirring periodically, or until the oats are soft and creamy.

3. Add the dried oregano, diced tomatoes, cooked sausage slices, salt, and pepper. Allow the flavors to combine and the food to heat through for a further two to three minutes.

4. Take the skillet off of the burner and pour the flavorful oatmeal onto a bowl for serving.

5. If wanted, garnish with grated Parmesan cheese and fresh basil leaves.

Nutritional Information (per serving):
- Calories: 320

- Total Fat: 15g
- Saturated Fat: 5g
- Cholesterol: 30mg
- Sodium: 450mg
- Total Carbohydrates: 30g
- Dietary Fiber: 5g
- Sugars: 2g
- Protein: 17g

Ingredient Substitutions:
- Use any variety of sausage you prefer, such as Italian, breakfast, or chorizo.
- Substitute diced sun-dried tomatoes for fresh tomatoes for a more intense flavor.
- Replace dried oregano with dried basil or thyme for a different herbal twist.

CHAPTER 3: REFRESHING BEVERAGE, SMOOTHIE AND JUICE RECIPES

Spinach Kale Smoothie

Prep Time: 5 minutes
Servings: 1

Ingredients:
- One tiny ripe banana, peeled and sliced
- One cup cleaned and raw spinach leaves
- One cup chopped and de stemmed kale leaves
- One-third cup plain Greek yogurt (unsweetened)
- ½ cup almond milk (or any other type of milk) without added sugar
- One spoonful of flaxseed meal
- One teaspoon of optional honey or maple syrup
- ½ teaspoon of pure vanilla extract
- Half a cup of ice cubes

Instructions
1. Start by getting your fresh ingredients ready. After giving the spinach leaves a good wash, destem the kale and slice it into little pieces.

2. Put the spinach, kale, Greek yogurt, sliced banana, ground flaxseeds, almond milk, vanilla extract, and honey or maple syrup (if using) in a blender.

3. Tightly fit the cover and process at high speed until the mixture is creamy and smooth, making sure all the components are well combined.

4. If the consistency is too thick, thin it up with a small amount of additional almond milk. If it's too thin, blend again after adding a few more ice cubes.

5. After the smoothie reaches the consistency you want, taste it and add additional honey or maple syrup to adjust the sweetness if needed.

6. Transfer the smoothie into a tall glass, top with a banana slice or a sprig of fresh mint, if preferred, and serve right away.

Nutritional Information (per serving):
- Calories: 180
- Carbohydrates: 30g
- Protein: 10g
- Fat: 4g
- Fiber: 7g

Strawberry Pineapple Smoothie

Prep Time: 5 minutes
Servings: 1

Ingredients:
- One cup fresh or frozen strawberries
- One cup of fresh or canned pineapple chunks
- 1 small ripe banana, peeled and sliced
- ½ cup plain Greek yogurt (unsweetened)
- ½ cup unsweetened coconut milk
- 1 tablespoon ground flaxseeds
- ½ teaspoon pure vanilla extract
- One teaspoon of optional honey or maple syrup
- ½ cup ice cubes

Instructions:
1. Hulling the strawberries and chopping the pineapple into bits will prepare the fresh ingredients.

2. Strawberries, pineapple chunks, banana slices, Greek yogurt, coconut milk, ground flaxseeds, vanilla extract, and honey or maple syrup (if used) should all be combined in a blender.

3. Make sure all the ingredients are completely incorporated, then tighten the cover and blend on high speed until the mixture is smooth and creamy.

4. If the consistency is too thick, add extra coconut milk; if it's too thin, add more ice cubes.

5. After tasting the smoothie, taste it and add extra honey or maple syrup to make it more sweet.

6. After the smoothie is perfectly smooth, pour it into glasses, top with a strawberry slice or a pineapple wedge, if you'd like, and serve right away.

Nutritional Information (per serving):
- Calories: 200
- Carbohydrates: 35g
- Protein: 8g
- Fat: 4g
- Fiber: 6g

Cherry Smoothie

Prep Time: 5 minutes
Servings: 1

Ingredients:
- One cup of pitted fresh or frozen cherries
- 1 small ripe banana, peeled and sliced
- ½ cup plain Greek yogurt (unsweetened)
- ½ cup unsweetened almond milk
- 1 tablespoon ground flaxseeds
- ½ teaspoon pure vanilla extract

- One teaspoon of optional honey or maple syrup
- ½ cup ice cubes

Instructions:

1. Pit the cherries using fresh cherries to begin the preparation process.

2. Put the sliced banana, Greek yogurt, almond milk, ground flaxseeds, pitted cherries, vanilla extract, and honey or maple syrup (if using) in a blender.

3. Tightly fit the cover and process at high speed until the mixture is creamy and smooth, making sure all the components are well combined.

4. If the smoothie is too thick, add more almond milk, and if it's too thin, add more ice cubes to adjust the consistency.

5. After tasting the smoothie, add more honey or maple syrup to taste and adjust sweetness as needed.

6. After the smoothie is well blended, pour it into glasses, top with a cherry if you'd like, and serve right away.

Nutritional Information (per serving):
- Calories: 180
- Carbohydrates: 30g
- Protein: 8g
- Fat: 4g
- Fiber: 5g

Mango Raspberry Smoothie

Prep Time: 5 minutes
Servings: 1

Ingredients:

- 1 cup frozen mango chunks
- 1/2 cup fresh or frozen raspberries
- 1 small ripe banana, peeled and sliced
- 1/2 cup plain Greek yogurt (unsweetened)
- 1/2 cup unsweetened almond milk
- 1 tablespoon ground flaxseeds
- 1/2 teaspoon pure vanilla extract
- One tablespoon of optional honey or maple syrup
- 1/2 cup ice cubes

Instructions:

1. Start by preparing the frozen mango chunks and rinsing the raspberries if using fresh ones.

2. In a blender, combine the frozen mango chunks, raspberries, sliced banana, Greek yogurt, almond milk, ground flaxseeds, vanilla extract, and honey or maple syrup (if using).

3. Tightly fit the cover and process at high speed until the mixture is creamy and smooth, making sure all the components are well combined

4. If the smoothie is too thick, add more almond milk, and if it's too thin, add more ice cubes to adjust the consistency.

5. Taste the smoothie and adjust sweetness as desired by adding more honey or maple syrup.

6. Once blended to perfection, pour the smoothie into glasses, garnish with a raspberry or mango slice if desired, and serve immediately.

Nutritional Information (per serving):
- Calories: 200
- Carbohydrates: 35g
- Protein: 8g
- Fat: 4g
- Fiber: 6g

Beet Carrot Pineapple Orange Juice

Prep Time: 10 minutes
Servings: 1

Ingredients:
- 1 small beet, peeled and chopped
- 1 medium carrot, peeled and chopped
- One cup of canned or fresh pineapple chunks
- Juice of 2 oranges
- 1/2 cup water
- One tablespoon of optional honey or maple syrup
- Ice cubes (optional)

Instructions:
1. Prepare the beet and carrot by peeling and chopping them into manageable pieces.

2. In a blender, combine the chopped beet, carrot, pineapple chunks, orange juice, water, and honey or maple syrup (if using).

3. Tightly fit the cover and process at high speed until the mixture is creamy and smooth, making sure all the components are well combined

4. If the smoothie is too thick, add more almond milk, and if it's too thin, add more ice cubes to adjust the consistency.

5. Taste the juice and adjust sweetness as desired by adding more honey or maple syrup.

6. Once blended to perfection, pour the juice into glasses, garnish with a slice of orange or a sprig of mint if desired, and serve immediately.

Nutritional Information (per serving):
- Calories: 120
- Carbohydrates: 30g

- Protein: 2g
- Fat: 0g
- Fiber: 5g

Celery Juice

Prep Time: 10 minutes
Servings: 1

Ingredients:
- 4-5 stalks of celery, trimmed and washed
- 1/2 cup water
- Juice of 1 lemon
- One teaspoon of optional honey or maple syrup
 - Ice cubes (optional)

Instructions:
1. After giving the celery stalks a thorough wash, cut off any rough ends.

2. Process the celery stalks in a juicer until they are fully juiced, producing a bright green liquid.

3. Pour the celery juice into a big glass or pitcher.

4. Stir thoroughly to blend the celery juice with water and one lemon's juice.

5. After tasting the juice, add honey or maple syrup to taste and adjust sweetness as needed.

6. Before serving, cool the juice by adding ice cubes, if preferred.

7. Transfer the celery juice into glasses, top with a slice of lemon or a celery stalk, if preferred, and serve right away.

Nutritional Information (per serving):
- Calories: 20
- Carbohydrates: 5g
- Protein: 1g
- Fat: 0g
- Fiber: 2g

Cucumber Green Juice

Prep Time: 10 minutes
Servings: 1

Ingredients:
- 1 large cucumber, washed and chopped
- 2 cups spinach leaves, washed
- 1 green apple, cored and chopped
- 1/2 cup water
- Juice of 1 lime
- One teaspoon of optional honey or maple syrup
- Ice cubes (optional)

Instructions:
1. Wash the cucumber thoroughly and chop it into chunks.

2. In a juicer, process the cucumber chunks, spinach leaves, and chopped green apple until they are completely juiced, yielding a vibrant green liquid.

3. Transfer the green juice to a pitcher or large glass.

4. Add water and the juice of one lime to the green juice, stirring well to combine.

5. After tasting the juice, add honey or maple syrup to taste and adjust sweetness as needed.

6. If desired, add ice cubes to the juice to chill it before serving.

7. Pour the cucumber green juice into glasses, garnish with a cucumber slice or lime wedge if desired, and serve immediately.

Nutritional Information (per serving):
- Calories: 60
- Carbohydrates: 15g
- Protein: 2g
- Fat: 0g
- Fiber: 4g

Citrus Splash

Prep Time: 5 minutes
Servings: 1

Ingredients:
- 2 oranges, peeled and segmented
- 1 grapefruit, peeled and segmented
- 1/2 cup water
- Ice cubes (optional)

Instructions:
1. Remove any seeds or pith by peeling and segmenting the grapefruit and oranges.

2. Place the orange and grapefruit segments in a blender or juicer and pulse until fully juiced, creating a bright orange drink.

3. Pour the juice into a big glass or pitcher.

4. Carefully whisk in the water after adding it to the juice.

5. Before serving, chill the juice by adding ice cubes, if preferred.

6. Transfer the orange-grapefruit juice into glasses; if preferred, top with an orange or grapefruit slice, and serve right away.

Nutritional Information (per serving):
- Calories: 80
- Carbohydrates: 20g
- Protein: 1g
- Fat: 0g
- Fiber: 4g

Cinnamon Iced Tea

Prep Time: 5 minutes
Cook Time: 15 minutes
Servings: 4

Ingredients:
- 2 cinnamon sticks
- 4 cups water
- 4 black tea bags
- Two teaspoon of optional honey or maple syrup
- Lemon slices or cinnamon sticks for garnish (optional)
- Ice cubes

Instructions:
1. Heat the water in a medium saucepan until it boils.

2. After the water reaches a boil, add the cinnamon sticks and turn down the heat. To absorb its flavor, let the cinnamon simmer in the water for five to ten minutes.

3. Take the pot off of the burner and put the bags of black tea in. As directed on the package, steep the tea bags in the water flavored with cinnamon for three to five minutes.

4. Take out the cinnamon sticks and tea bags from the saucepan and allow the tea to come to room temperature.

5. After the tea has cooled, pour it into a pitcher and chill it.

6. Transfer the cold cinnamon iced tea into ice cube-filled glasses when ready to serve.

7. You can add honey or maple syrup to the tea if you'd like, stirring until dissolved.

8. Garnish each glass with a lemon slice or cinnamon stick for added flair, and enjoy!

Nutritional Information (per serving, without sweetener):
- Calories: 0
- Carbohydrates: 0g
- Protein: 0g
- Fat: 0g
- Fiber: 0g

Ingredient Substitutions:
- Black Tea Bags: Green tea bags or herbal tea bags can be substituted for black tea if preferred.

CHAPTER 4: LUNCH- SALAD RECIPES

Potato Bean Salad with Herb Dressing

Prep Time: 15 minutes
Cook Time: 15 minutes
Serving : 4

Salad:

- 2 cups baby potatoes, halved (substitution: sweet potatoes or cauliflower florets)
- One can of 15 oz kidney beans, rinsed and drained (substitution: chickpeas, black beans, or cannellini beans)
- One cup of green beans, trimmed and cut into small pieces
- 1/4 cup red onion, finely diced
- 1/4 cup celery, thinly sliced
- 1/4 cup fresh parsley, chopped (substitution: 1 tablespoon dried parsley)
- Salt and pepper to taste

Herb Dressing:
- 1/4 cup extra virgin olive oil
- 2 tablespoons apple cider vinegar
- 1 tablespoon lemon juice
- 1 clove garlic, minced
- 1 teaspoon Dijon mustard
- One tablespoon of honey or maple syrup (optional, substitution: agave nectar)
- 2 tablespoons fresh chives, chopped (substitution: 1 tablespoon dried chives)
- 2 tablespoons fresh dill, chopped (substitution: 1 tablespoon dried dill)
- Salt and pepper to taste

Instructions:

1. Start by getting the baby potatoes ready. Transfer them to a boiling pot of salted water. Simmer for ten to twelve minutes, or until soft but not mushy. After draining, allow it to cool somewhat.

2. Blanch the green beans in boiling water for two to three minutes, then stop the cooking by transferring them to a bowl of ice water while the potatoes are cooking. After draining, set away.

3. Place the blanched green beans, diced red onion, sliced celery, cooked baby potatoes, kidney beans (or your favorite substitute), and chopped parsley (or dried parsley) in a big salad dish. To taste, add salt and pepper for seasoning.

4. In order to make the herb dressing, combine the extra virgin olive oil, lemon juice, apple cider vinegar, minced garlic, Dijon mustard, and honey or maple syrup (if desired; agave nectar can be used in its place) in a small bowl. Add the chopped dill and chives (or dried dill, if preferred). To taste, add salt and pepper for seasoning.

5. Drizzle the salad with the herb dressing and gently toss to cover all of the ingredients.

6. Before serving, let the flavors mingle for a few minutes. If desired, garnish with extra finely chopped herbs.

Nutritional Information (per serving):
- Calories: 220 kcal
- Total Fat: 10g
  - Saturated Fat: 1.5g
  - Trans Fat: 0g
- Cholesterol: 0mg
- Sodium: 180mg
- Total Carbohydrates: 28g
  - Dietary Fiber: 6g
  - Sugars: 3g
- Protein: 6g

Creamy Pesto Chicken Salad with Greens

Prep Time: 15 minutes
Cook Time: 0 minutes
Servings: 4

Salad:
- Two cups cooked diced chicken breast,
- 4 cups mixed salad greens (such as spinach, arugula, and romaine lettuce)
- 1/2 cup cherry tomatoes, halved
- 1/4 cup cucumber, thinly sliced
- 1/4 cup of diced red bell pepper,
- 1/4 cup red onion, thinly sliced
- Salt and pepper to taste

Creamy Pesto Dressing:
- 1/4 cup plain Greek yogurt
- 2 tablespoons prepared basil pesto
- 1 tablespoon lemon juice
- 1 clove garlic, minced
- Salt and pepper to taste

Instructions:
1. The cooked chicken breast, mixed salad greens, cherry tomatoes, cucumber, red bell pepper, and red onion should all be combined in a big salad dish. To taste, add salt and pepper for seasoning.

2. Combine the plain Greek yogurt, basil pesto, lemon juice, and minced garlic in a separate bowl to make the creamy pesto dressing. To taste, add salt and pepper for seasoning.

3. Drizzle the salad with the velvety pesto dressing, gently tossing to coat all of the ingredients.

4. Before serving, let the flavors mingle for a few minutes.

5. Spoon the salad onto bowls or serving trays.

6. Optional: Garnish with additional basil leaves or grated Parmesan cheese for extra flavor and visual appeal.

Nutritional Information (per serving):
- Calories: 250 kcal
- Total Fat: 12g
  - Saturated Fat: 2g
  - Trans Fat: 0g
- Cholesterol: 70mg
- Sodium: 350mg
- Total Carbohydrates: 7g
  - Dietary Fiber: 2g
  - Sugars: 3g
- Protein: 28g

Spinach Salad with Raspberries and Candied Walnuts

Prep Time: 15 minutes
Cook Time: 10 minutes
Servings: 4

Salad:
- Four cup of fresh spinach leaves, washed and dried
- 1 cup fresh raspberries
- 1/4 cup red onion, thinly sliced
- 1/4 cup crumbled feta cheese (optional)
- Salt and pepper to taste

Candied Walnuts:
- 1/2 cup walnuts
- 2 tablespoons granulated sugar (substitution: sugar-free sweetener)
- 1 tablespoon water

Balsamic Vinaigrette:
- 2 tablespoons extra virgin olive oil
- 1 tablespoon balsamic vinegar
- 1 teaspoon Dijon mustard
- 1/2 teaspoon honey or maple syrup (optional, substitution: sugar-free sweetener)
- Salt and pepper to taste

Instructions:
1. Prepare the candied walnuts first. Put the walnuts, water, and granulated sugar (or sugar-free sweetener) in a small skillet over medium heat. Stir the sugar continuously until it melts and forms a caramelized coating over the walnuts. To cool and solidify, move the candied walnuts to a baking sheet covered with parchment.

2. Place the raspberries, finely sliced red onion, crumbled feta cheese (if using), and fresh spinach leaves in a large salad bowl. To taste, add salt and pepper for seasoning.

3. In a small bowl, mix the extra virgin olive oil, balsamic vinegar, Dijon mustard, honey or maple syrup (if using, or use sugar-free sweetener in its place) to make the balsamic vinaigrette. To taste, add salt and pepper for seasoning.

4. Toss the salad mixture carefully to coat all the ingredients after drizzling it with the balsamic vinaigrette

5. Break the candied walnuts into smaller pieces and sprinkle them over the salad just before serving, to maintain their crunchy texture.

6. Optional: Garnish with a few additional raspberries and a sprinkle of freshly ground black pepper for an extra burst of flavor and visual appeal.

Nutritional Information (per serving):
- Calories: 180 kcal
- Total Fat: 14g
  - Saturated Fat: 2g
  - Trans Fat: 0g
- Cholesterol: 5mg
- Sodium: 120mg
- Total Carbohydrates: 10g
  - Dietary Fiber: 3g
  - Sugars: 5g
- Protein: 4g

Ruby Raspberry Slaw

Prep Time: 10 minutes
Cook Time: 0 minutes
Servings: 4

Slaw:
- 3 cups shredded red cabbage
- 1 cup shredded carrots
- 1 cup fresh raspberries
- 1/4 cup red onion, thinly sliced
- Two tablespoon of optional chopped fresh mint leaves
- Salt and pepper to taste

Dressing:
- 2 tablespoons extra virgin olive oil
- 1 tablespoon apple cider vinegar
- 1 tablespoon lemon juice
- One tablespoon of optional honey or maple syrup substitution: sugar-free sweetener)
- 1/2 teaspoon Dijon mustard

- Salt and pepper to taste

Instructions:

1. Combine the shredded red cabbage, shredded carrots, fresh raspberries, thinly sliced red onion, and chopped fresh mint leaves (if using) in a large bowl. To taste, add salt and pepper for seasoning.

2. To prepare the dressing, whisk together the extra virgin olive oil, apple cider vinegar, lemon juice, honey or maple syrup (if using, or substitution with sugar-free sweetener), and Dijon mustard in a small bowl. To taste, add salt and pepper for seasoning.

3. Toss the salad mixture carefully to coat all the ingredients after drizzling it with the dressing.

4. Allow the flavors to meld together for a few minutes before serving, allowing the raspberries to release their natural juices and infuse the slaw with their sweet flavor.

5. Optional: Garnish with additional fresh raspberries and mint leaves for an extra burst of color and freshness.

Nutritional Information (per serving):
- Calories: 120 kcal
- Total Fat: 7g
  - Saturated Fat: 1g
  - Trans Fat: 0g
- Cholesterol: 0mg
- Sodium: 60mg
- Total Carbohydrates: 15g
  - Dietary Fiber: 5g
  - Sugars: 8g
- Protein: 2g

Watermelon Salad with Coconut Rice

Prep Time: 15 minutes
Cook Time: 20 minutes
Servings: 4

Salad:
- 2 cups cooked brown rice (substitution: cauliflower rice for lower carbohydrate option)
- 2 cups diced watermelon
- 1/4 cup shredded unsweetened coconut
- 1/4 cup chopped fresh cilantro
- 1/4 cup red bell pepper, diced
- 1/4 cup red onion, thinly sliced
- Salt and pepper to taste

Dressing:
- 2 tablespoons lime juice
- 1 tablespoon extra virgin olive oil
- One tablespoon of optional honey or maple syrup (optional, substitution: sugar-free sweetener)
- 1/2 teaspoon ground cumin
- Salt and pepper to taste

Instructions:
1. Combine the cooked brown rice (or cauliflower rice), diced watermelon, shredded unsweetened coconut, chopped fresh cilantro, diced red bell pepper, and thinly sliced red onion in a large mixing bowl. To taste, add salt and pepper for seasoning.

2. To prepare the dressing, whisk together the lime juice, extra virgin olive oil, honey or maple syrup (if using, or substitution with sugar-free sweetener), ground cumin, salt, and pepper in a small bowl.

3. Toss the salad mixture carefully to coat all the ingredients after drizzling it with the dressing.

4. Allow the flavors to meld together for a few minutes before serving, allowing the sweetness of the watermelon and the tropical aroma of coconut to infuse the salad.

5. Optional: Garnish with additional fresh cilantro leaves and a sprinkle of shredded coconut for an extra burst of flavor and visual appeal.

Nutritional Information (per serving):
- Calories: 180 kcal
- Total Fat: 6g
  - Saturated Fat: 3g
  - Trans Fat: 0g
- Cholesterol: 0mg
- Sodium: 80mg
- Total Carbohydrates: 29g
  - Dietary Fiber: 3g
  - Sugars: 8g
- Protein: 3g

Mixed Greens with Lentils & Sliced Apple

Prep Time: 15 minutes
Cook Time: 20 minutes
Servings: 4

Salad:
- 4 cups mixed salad greens (such as spinach, arugula, and mesclun)
- 1 cup cooked lentils (substitution: canned lentils, drained and rinsed)
- 1 medium apple, thinly sliced (any variety of your choice)
- 1/4 cup red onion, thinly sliced
- 1/4 cup chopped walnuts (optional)

- Salt and pepper to taste

Dressing:
- 2 tablespoons extra virgin olive oil
- 1 tablespoon apple cider vinegar
- 1 teaspoon Dijon mustard
- 1/2 teaspoon honey or maple syrup (optional, substitution: sugar-free sweetener)
- Salt and pepper to taste

Instructions:
1. Combine the mixed salad greens, cooked lentils (or canned lentils), thinly sliced apple, thinly sliced red onion, and chopped walnuts (if using) in a large salad bowl. To taste, add salt and pepper for seasoning.

2. To prepare the dressing, whisk together the extra virgin olive oil, apple cider vinegar, Dijon mustard, honey or maple syrup (if using, or substitution with sugar-free sweetener), salt, and pepper in a small bowl.

3. Toss the salad mixture carefully to coat all the ingredients after drizzling it with the dressing

4. Allow the flavors to meld together for a few minutes before serving, allowing the sweetness of the apple and the nuttiness of the lentils to complement the freshness of the mixed greens.

5. Optional: Garnish with additional chopped walnuts and a sprinkle of freshly ground black pepper for an extra burst of flavor and texture.

Nutritional Information (per serving):
- Calories: 220 kcal
- Total Fat: 12g
  - Saturated Fat: 1.5g
  - Trans Fat: 0g
- Cholesterol: 0mg
- Sodium: 150mg
- Total Carbohydrates: 24g

- Dietary Fiber: 6g
 - Sugars: 9g
- Protein: 7g

Avocado Egg Salad

Prep Time: 10 minutes
Cook Time: 10 minutes
Servings: 4

Salad:
- Two ripe avocado, diced
- 4 hard-boiled eggs, chopped
- 1/4 cup red onion, finely diced
- 1/4 cup celery, thinly sliced
- 2 tablespoons chopped fresh cilantro or parsley
- Salt and pepper to taste

Dressing:
- 2 tablespoons plain Greek yogurt
- 1 tablespoon lemon juice
- 1 teaspoon Dijon mustard
- Salt and pepper to taste

Instructions:
1. Combine the diced avocados, chopped hard-boiled eggs, finely diced red onion, thinly sliced celery, and chopped fresh cilantro or parsley in a large salad bowl. To taste, add salt and pepper for seasoning.

2. To prepare the dressing, whisk together the plain Greek yogurt, lemon juice, Dijon mustard, salt, and pepper in a small bowl.

3. Toss the salad mixture carefully to coat all the ingredients after drizzling it with the dressing

4. Allow the flavors to meld together for a few minutes before serving, allowing the creamy richness of avocado and the savory goodness of eggs to shine through.

5. Optional: Garnish with additional chopped cilantro or parsley for an extra burst of freshness and color.

Nutritional Information (per serving):
- Calories: 220 kcal
- Total Fat: 16g
  - Saturated Fat: 3.5g
  - Trans Fat: 0g
- Cholesterol: 215mg
- Sodium: 150mg
- Total Carbohydrates: 11g
  - Dietary Fiber: 7g
  - Sugars: 2g
- Protein: 10g

Sesame-Garlic Spinach Salad

Prep Time: 10 minutes
Cook Time: 5 minutes
Servings: 4

Salad:
- Six cups fresh spinach leaves, washed and dried
- 1/4 cup sliced almonds, toasted
- 2 tablespoons sesame seeds, toasted
- 1/4 cup red bell pepper, thinly sliced
- 2 green onions, thinly sliced
- Salt and pepper to taste

Sesame-Garlic Dressing:
- 2 tablespoons sesame oil

- 1 tablespoon low-sodium soy sauce (substitution: tamari for gluten-free option)
- 1 tablespoon rice vinegar
- 1 clove garlic, minced
- 1/2 teaspoon honey or maple syrup (optional, substitution: sugar-free sweetener)
- 1/2 teaspoon grated fresh ginger (optional)
- Salt and pepper to taste

Instructions:

1. Combine the fresh spinach leaves, toasted sliced almonds, toasted sesame seeds, thinly sliced red bell pepper, and sliced green onions in a large bowl. To taste, add salt and pepper for seasoning.

2. To prepare the sesame-garlic dressing, whisk together the sesame oil, low-sodium soy sauce (or tamari), rice vinegar, minced garlic, honey or maple syrup (if using, or substitution with sugar-free sweetener), grated fresh ginger (if using), salt, and pepper in a small bowl.

3. Toss the salad mixture carefully to coat all the ingredients after drizzling it with the dressing

4. Allow the flavors to meld together for a few minutes before serving, allowing the sesame and garlic flavors to infuse the salad.

5. Optional: Garnish with additional toasted sesame seeds and sliced green onions for an extra burst of flavor and texture.

Nutritional Information (per serving):
- Calories: 180 kcal
- Total Fat: 14g
  - Saturated Fat: 2g
  - Trans Fat: 0g
- Cholesterol: 0mg
- Sodium: 250mg
- Total Carbohydrates: 9g
  - Dietary Fiber: 4g

  - Sugars: 2g
  - Protein: 6g

CHAPTER 5: LUNCH- TASTY SOUP RECIPES

French Lentil Carrot Soup

Prep Time: 10 minutes
Cook Time: 30 minutes
Servings: 4

Ingredients

- 1 cup French lentils, rinsed
- 2 tablespoons olive oil
- 1 onion, finely chopped
- 2 cloves garlic, minced
- 3 carrots, peeled and diced
- 1 celery stalk, diced
- 1 teaspoon ground cumin
- 1/2 teaspoon ground turmeric
- 1/2 teaspoon dried thyme
- 6 cups low-sodium vegetable broth
- Salt and pepper, to taste
- Fresh parsley or cilantro, chopped (for garnish)

Instructions

1. Two cups of water should be brought to a boil in a medium saucepan. After rinsing, add the lentils and boil until they are cooked, 15 to 20 minutes. After draining, set away.

2. Heat the olive oil in a big saucepan or Dutch oven over medium heat. When the onion is tender, add it and sauté it for three to four minutes. Add the minced garlic and simmer for a further minute after stirring.

3. Include the chopped celery and carrots in the pot. Add the ground thyme, turmeric, and cumin.

4. Add the vegetable broth with low sodium and boil the mixture. Cook the carrots for 20 to 25 minutes, or until they are soft.

5. For a smoother texture, use an immersion blender to purée a portion of the soup directly in the pot until desired consistency is reached. Alternatively, carefully transfer a portion of the soup to a blender and blend until smooth, then return to the pot.

6. Stir in the cooked lentils and simmer for an additional 5-10 minutes to blend the flavors. Season with salt and pepper to taste. Serve

Nutritional Information (per serving)
- Calories: 220
- Total Fat: 7g
  - Saturated Fat: 1g
- Cholesterol: 0mg
- Sodium: 480mg
- Total Carbohydrates: 31g
  - Dietary Fiber: 9g
  - Sugars: 5g
- Protein: 10g

Beefy cabbage bean stew

Prep Time: 15 minutes
Cook Time: 1 hour 15 minutes
Servings: 6

Ingredients
- 1 pound lean beef stew meat, cut into small pieces

- 1 tablespoon olive oil
- 1 onion, finely chopped
- 2 cloves garlic, minced
- 3 cups green cabbage, thinly sliced
- 2 carrots, peeled and diced
- 1 celery stalk, diced
- One can of 14.5 ounce low-sodium diced tomatoes
- 4 cups low-sodium beef broth
- 1 teaspoon dried thyme
- 1 teaspoon paprika
- 1/2 teaspoon black pepper
- One can of 15 ounces low-sodium kidney beans, rinsed and drained
- Salt, to taste
- Fresh parsley, chopped (for garnish)

Instructions

1. Heat the olive oil in a big pot or Dutch oven over medium heat. Add the beef stew meat and simmer for 5 to 7 minutes, or until browned all over. Set the steak aside after taking it out of the pot

2. Add the chopped onion to the same saucepan and sauté it for 3–4 minutes, or until it becomes tender. One more minute is spent cooking after adding the minced garlic.

3. Add the diced carrots, celery, and sliced cabbage. Cook until the vegetables begin to soften, about 5 to 7 minutes. Incorporate the paprika, black pepper, and dried thyme, mixing thoroughly.

4. Add low-sodium beef broth and diced tomatoes with their juices. Put the browned steak back in the saucepan. After bringing the stew to a simmer, turn down the heat. After 45 to 60 minutes of simmering, stirring now and again, the meat should be soft and the flavors should blend.

5. Add the kidney beans and cook for a further 10 to 15 minutes, or until the beans are thoroughly heated. Add salt to taste and season.

Nutritional Information (per serving)

- Calories: 280
- Total Fat: 8g
  - Saturated Fat: 2g
- Cholesterol: 45mg
- Sodium: 380mg
- Total Carbohydrates: 26g
  - Dietary Fiber: 7g
  - Sugars: 6g
- Protein: 26g

Ingredient Substitutions
- Substitute with lean ground beef or turkey if preferred.
- Use vegetable broth for a vegetarian option.
- Cannellini beans or black beans can be used as alternatives.

Tips
- For added convenience, prepare this stew in a slow cooker. Brown the beef and sauté the aromatics before transferring everything to the slow cooker and cooking on low for 6-8 hours.
- This stew can be stored in the refrigerator for up to 3 days or frozen for longer storage. Warm it on a stovetop or in the microwave before serving.

Hazelnut Asparagus Soup

Prep Time: 10 minutes
Cook Time: 25 minutes
Servings: 4

Ingredients
- 1 pound asparagus, tough ends trimmed and chopped
- 1 tablespoon olive oil
- 1 onion, chopped
- 2 cloves garlic, minced
- 4 cups low-sodium vegetable broth
- 1/2 cup roasted hazelnuts, skins removed

- Salt and pepper, to taste
- Fresh lemon juice, for serving (optional)
- Fresh chives, chopped (for garnish)

Instructions

1. Heat the olive oil in a big pot or Dutch oven over medium heat. Add chopped onion and cook until softened, about 3 to 4 minutes. Saute the chopped asparagus and minced garlic for a further two to three minutes.

2. Add the vegetable broth with low sodium content and boil the mixture. Once the asparagus is tender, cook it in the covered pot for 15 to 20 minutes.

3. Pour the soup into a blender or purée it with an immersion blender until it's smooth. When combining hot liquids, exercise caution.

4. Pulse the toasted hazelnuts in a food processor or blender until they are finely crushed.

5. Blend the soup and mix in the ground hazelnuts. This will give the soup a deliciously creamy texture and nuttiness.

6. Add salt and pepper to taste and season. Add a squeeze of fresh lemon juice if desired.

Nutritional Information (per serving)

- Calories: 180
- Total Fat: 12g
  - Saturated Fat: 1g
- Cholesterol: 0mg
- Sodium: 380mg
- Total Carbohydrates: 15g
  - Dietary Fiber: 5g
  - Sugars: 5g
- Protein: 6g

Tips

- To enhance the soup's creaminess without adding dairy, incorporate a small amount of unsweetened almond milk or coconut milk.
- Serve this soup as a light starter or pair it with a salad or whole-grain bread for a complete meal.

Salmon Dill Soup

Prep Time: 15 minutes
Cook Time: 25 minutes
Servings: 4

Ingredients
- 1 tablespoon olive oil
- 1 onion, finely chopped
- 2 cloves garlic, minced
- 3 cups low-sodium vegetable broth
- 1 cup water
- 2 medium potatoes, peeled and diced
- 2 carrots, peeled and diced
- 1 celery stalk, diced
- 1 teaspoon dried dill weed
- 1/2 teaspoon dried thyme
- 1/2 teaspoon black pepper
- 1/2 pound fresh salmon filet, skin removed and diced
- One cup of unsweetened or low fat almond milk
- Salt, to taste
- Fresh dill, chopped (for garnish)
- Lemon wedges (optional, for serving)

Instructions
1. Heat the olive oil in a big pot or Dutch oven over medium heat. Add chopped onion and cook until softened, about 3 to 4 minutes. Cook the minced garlic for a further one to two minutes.

2. Add water and the low-sodium vegetable broth. To the pot, add the diced potatoes, carrots, and celery. Add dried dill weed, black pepper, and thyme for seasoning. Simmer the mixture for 15 to 20 minutes, or until the vegetables are soft.

3. Add the chopped salmon filet and mix gently. Let the salmon cook for a further five to seven minutes, or until it is well cooked and flakes readily with a fork.

4. Add the unsweetened almond milk or low-fat milk and whisk just until combined. After two to three minutes, let the soup simmer to reheat.

5. Add freshly cut parsley as a garnish.

Nutritional Information (per serving)
- Calories: 250
- Total Fat: 8g
  - Saturated Fat: 1.5g
- Cholesterol: 35mg
- Sodium: 380mg
- Total Carbohydrates: 25g
  - Dietary Fiber: 3g
  - Sugars: 5g
- Protein: 20g

Ingredient Substitutions
- Salmon: Substitute with canned salmon or trout if fresh salmon is not available.
- Low-Fat Milk: Use unsweetened almond milk or soy milk for a dairy-free option.

Turkey Sausage and Lentil Soup

Prep Time: 15 minutes

Cook Time: 30 minutes

Servings: 6

Ingredients

- 1 tablespoon olive oil
- 1 onion, finely chopped
- 2 cloves garlic, minced
- 2 carrots, peeled and diced
- 2 celery stalks, diced
- 8 ounces turkey sausage, casings removed and crumbled
- 1 cup dried brown lentils, rinsed
- 6 cups low-sodium chicken broth
- 1 teaspoon dried thyme
- 1/2 teaspoon smoked paprika
- Salt and pepper, to taste
- Fresh parsley, chopped (for garnish)

Instructions

1. Heat the olive oil in a big pot or Dutch oven over medium heat. Add chopped onion and cook until softened, about 3 to 4 minutes. Cook the minced garlic for a further one to two minutes.

2. Include the turkey sausage crumbles in the saucepan. Cook for 5 to 7 minutes, breaking up the meat with a spoon, or until it's browned and well done.

3. Add the chopped celery and carrots. Simmer the vegetables for a further three to four minutes, or until they begin to soften. Fill the pot with the washed lentils.

4. Add the chicken broth with minimal sodium content. Add smoked paprika and dried thyme for seasoning. The lentils should be soft after 25 to 30 minutes of simmering the mixture.

5. Add freshly cut parsley as a garnish.

Nutritional Information (per serving)

- Calories: 280

- Total Fat: 9g
  - Saturated Fat: 2g
- Cholesterol: 35mg
- Sodium: 380mg
- Total Carbohydrates: 30g
  - Dietary Fiber: 12g
  - Sugars: 4g
- Protein: 20g

Ingredient Substitutions
- Turkey Sausage: Substitute with chicken or pork sausage if preferred, opting for lean varieties.
- Brown Lentils: Green or red lentils can be used as alternatives.

CHAPTER 6: LUNCH- BEAN, RICE AND PASTA RECIPES

Kale Soup with Turkey and Beans

Prep Time: 15 minutes
Cook Time: 30 minutes
Servings: 6

Ingredients:
- 1 tbsp of extra virgin olive oil
- 1 finely chopped onion
- 2 minced garlic cloves
- 2 sliced carrots, skin removed
- 2 sliced stalks of celery
- 8 oz of diced, skinless turkey breast
- 6 cups of chicken broth with reduced sodium
- 1 can (15 oz) of chopped tomatoes, juice included
- 2 cups of kale, chopped and de-stemmed
- 1 can (15 oz) of rinsed and drained low-sodium kidney beans
- 1 tsp of dried thyme
- 1 tsp of dried oregano
- Salt and pepper

Instructions

1. Start by warming up the olive oil in a big pot over a medium flame. Toss in the chopped onion and let it cook until it's clear and soft, which should take about 5 minutes. Now, stir in the garlic for another minute, making sure it doesn't burn.

2. Next, it's time for the carrots and celery. Throw them into the pot and give them about 5 minutes to cook, stirring here and there, until they're starting to get tender.

3. Now, add the turkey pieces and cook them until they're nicely browned all around, which should be roughly 5 minutes.

4. Pour in the chicken broth and the tomatoes with all their juices. Let this all come to a gentle simmer and leave it be for 15 minutes to let all those delicious flavors come together.

5. It's kale and bean time! Add the kale, kidney beans, thyme, and oregano into the mix. Add salt and pepper to taste. Let the whole thing simmer for another 10 minutes, or until the kale has softened up.

Nutritional Information (per serving):
- Calories: 220
- Total Fat: 4g
- Saturated Fat: 1g
- Cholesterol: 35mg
- Sodium: 420mg
- Total Carbohydrates: 24g
- Dietary Fiber: 6g
- Sugars: 4g
- Protein: 22g

Ingredient Substitutions:
- For a vegetarian option, replace the turkey with additional beans or tofu.
- For a gluten-free option, ensure all ingredients, including the chicken broth and canned tomatoes, are labeled gluten-free.

Wholesome Barley and Mushroom Pilaf

Prep Time: 10 minutes

Cook Time: 40 minutes

Servings: 4

Ingredients:
- One cup of rinsed and drained pearl barley
- 2 cups low-sodium vegetable broth
- 1 tablespoon olive oil
- 1 onion, diced
- 2 cloves garlic, minced
- 8 ounces cremini mushrooms, sliced
- 1 teaspoon dried thyme
- 1 teaspoon dried rosemary
- Salt and black pepper to taste
- 1/4 cup chopped fresh parsley, for garnish

Instructions:

1. Grab a saucepan of medium size and toss in your washed pearl barley along with some low-sodium veggie stock. Crank up the heat to medium-high until it bubbles, then drop it down to a gentle simmer.

2. Slap a lid on it and let it do its thing for about half an hour to thirty-five minutes, just until it barely gets nice and soft and drinks up all the liquid. Then, kill the heat and let it chill undercover for a quick five.

3. Meanwhile, as your barley's getting all cozy, get some olive oil warming in a big pan over a medium flame. Chuck in your chopped onions and let them get all see-through and sweet, should take around five minutes.

4. Toss in the garlic and give it a quick minute, keeping things moving so it doesn't get too toasty.

5. Next up, slide those cremini mushroom slices into the pan and give them a good stir now and then. You want them to get a lovely golden color and become perfectly soft, which'll take you about 8 to 10 minutes.

6. Once those mushrooms are looking just right, it's time to bring the barley back into the mix. Dump it into the pan with the mushrooms, and sprinkle in your thyme and rosemary.

7. Mix it all up and let it get nice and hot together, which should be about 3 to 4 minutes. Hit it with a pinch of salt and pepper, just go by what your taste buds tell you.

8. Finally, scoop that hearty barley and mushroom pilaf into your favorite serving bowl and make it pretty with a handful of fresh parsley on top.

Nutritional Information (per serving):
- Calories: 220
- Total Fat: 4g
- Saturated Fat: 0.5g
- Cholesterol: 0mg
- Sodium: 240mg
- Total Carbohydrates: 40g
- Dietary Fiber: 8g
- Sugars: 2g
- Protein: 7g

Ingredient Substitutions:
- For a gluten-free option, substitute barley with quinoa or brown rice.
- Customize the pilaf by adding additional vegetables such as bell peppers, spinach, or peas according to personal preference and dietary needs.
- For added protein, incorporate cooked chickpeas or diced tofu into the pilaf.

Sesame-Garlic Beef & Broccoli with Whole-Wheat Noodles

Prep Time: 15 minutes
Cook Time: 20 minutes

Ingredients:
- 8 ounces whole-wheat spaghetti or noodles
- 1 pound lean beef steak, thinly sliced
- 2 tablespoons low-sodium soy sauce
- 1 tablespoon sesame oil
- 2 cloves garlic, minced
- 1 teaspoon grated fresh ginger
- 1 tablespoon olive oil
- 2 cups broccoli florets
- 1 red bell pepper, thinly sliced
- 2 green onions, chopped, for garnish
- Sesame seeds, for garnish

Instructions:
1. First things first, let's get that whole-wheat spaghetti or your choice of noodles bubbling away just like the box says, until they're perfectly al dente. Once they're done, give them a good drain and pop them to the side for later.

2. Now, grab a bowl and let's get that beef steak, sliced nice and thin, all cozy with a splash of low-sodium soy sauce, a drizzle of sesame oil, a bit of minced garlic, and a sprinkle of freshly grated ginger. Give it all a good mix to make sure the beef is lovingly coated, and let it chill out for a 10-minute marinade session.

3. Time to crank up the heat! Get your skillet nice and hot with a little olive oil over a medium-high flame. Toss in the beef that's been soaking up all those flavors and give it a quick sizzle for about 2-3 minutes, just until it's got a nice brown sear and is cooked just right. Scoop it out and let it hang out on the side.

4. Don't let that skillet cool down yet! Throw in the broccoli florets and some vibrant slices of red bell pepper. Give them a stir and cook for another 4-5 minutes until they're tender but still have that satisfying crunch.

5. It's reunion time! Bring the beef back into the skillet party with the veggies. Now, add in the whole-wheat spaghetti or noodles you set aside earlier, and toss

everything together like they're old friends catching up. You want every strand and piece to be warm and mingling with all those flavors.

6. Don't forget to sprinkle some chopped green onions and sesame seeds on top!

Nutritional Information (per serving):
- Calories: 380
- Total Fat: 12g
- Saturated Fat: 3g
- Cholesterol: 60mg
- Sodium: 420mg
- Total Carbohydrates: 38g
- Dietary Fiber: 7g
- Sugars: 4g
- Protein: 30g

Ingredient Substitutions:
- For a vegetarian option, substitute the beef steak with tofu or tempeh.
- If whole-wheat noodles are not available, you can use regular whole-wheat spaghetti or any other whole-grain pasta of your choice.

Spaghetti Bolognese

Prep Time: 15 minutes
Cook Time: 30 minutes
Servings: 4

Ingredients:
- 8 ounces whole-wheat spaghetti
- 1 tablespoon olive oil
- 1 onion, finely chopped
- 2 cloves garlic, minced
- 1 pound lean ground turkey
- 1 can (14.5 ounces) diced tomatoes, undrained
- 1 can (6 ounces) tomato paste

- 1 teaspoon dried basil
- 1 teaspoon dried oregano
- Salt and black pepper to taste
- Grated Parmesan cheese, for serving (optional)
- Chopped fresh basil, for garnish (optional)

Instructions:

1. As directed on the package, cook the whole-wheat spaghetti until it's al dente. After draining, set away.

2. Heat the olive oil in a big skillet over medium heat. Cook the minced garlic and finely diced onion for five minutes, or until the ingredients are tender.

3. After adding the lean ground turkey to the skillet, heat it for 8 to 10 minutes, breaking it up with a spoon, until it is browned and cooked through.

4. Add the tomato paste, dried oregano, dried basil, and chopped tomatoes together with their liquids. To taste, add salt and black pepper for seasoning. To enable the flavors to mingle, bring the sauce to a simmer and cook, stirring regularly, for 10 to 15 minutes.

5. Add the cooked whole-wheat after the sauce is finished. Distribute the sauce evenly over the spaghetti

6. If desired, Serve hot, garnished with grated Parmesan cheese and chopped fresh basil, if desired.

Nutritional Information (per serving):
- Calories: 350
- Total Fat: 9g
- Saturated Fat: 2g
- Cholesterol: 55mg
- Sodium: 480mg
- Total Carbohydrates: 45g
- Dietary Fiber: 8g
- Sugars: 10g
- Protein: 25g

- For a vegetarian option, substitute the lean ground turkey with cooked lentils or crumbled tofu.

CHAPTER 7: LUNCH- VEGETARIAN RECIPES

Grilled Eggplant and Portobello Mushroom Sandwich

Ingredients:
- 1 medium eggplant, sliced into 1/2-inch rounds
- 2 large portobello mushrooms, stems removed
- 2 tablespoons olive oil
- 2 cloves garlic, minced
- 1 teaspoon dried oregano
- Salt and black pepper to taste
- 4 whole grain burger buns or sandwich rolls
- 1 cup baby spinach leaves
- 1 large tomato, sliced
- 1/2 cup crumbled feta cheese (optional)
- Balsamic glaze (optional, for drizzling)

Instructions:
1. Turn the heat up to medium-high on the grill or grill pan.

2. Combine the olive oil, minced garlic, dried oregano, salt, and black pepper in a bowl to create a marinade.

3. Brush both sides of the eggplant slices and portobello mushrooms with the marinade.

4. Place the eggplant slices and portobello mushrooms on the preheated grill. Cook until they are cooked and have grill marks, about 4–5 minutes 3 per side.

5. While the vegetables are grilling, lightly toast the burger buns or sandwich rolls on the grill until they are warm and slightly crispy.

6. Assemble the sandwiches by placing a few spinach leaves on the bottom half of each bun, followed by a grilled portobello mushroom cap, grilled eggplant slices, tomato slices, and crumbled feta cheese (if using).

7. Drizzle each sandwich with a little balsamic glaze, if desired, and then top with the remaining half of the bun. Enjoy!

Nutritional Information (per serving):
- Calories: 290 kcal
- Carbohydrates: 37 g
- Protein: 10 g
- Fat: 13 g
- Fiber: 8 g
- Sodium: 530 mg

Quinoa and Vegetable Salad with Lemon Vinaigrette

Ingredients:
- 1 cup quinoa, rinsed
- 2 cups water or vegetable broth
- 1 cup cherry tomatoes, halved
- 1 cucumber, diced
- 1 diced bell pepper any color
- 1/4 cup red onion, finely chopped
- 1/4 cup fresh parsley, chopped

- 1/4 cup fresh mint leaves, chopped (optional)
- 1/4 cup crumbled feta cheese (optional)
- Salt and black pepper to taste

For the Lemon Vinaigrette:
- 1/4 cup extra virgin olive oil
- 2 tablespoons fresh lemon juice
- 1 teaspoon Dijon mustard
- 1 clove garlic, minced
- One teaspoon of optional honey or maple syrup
- Salt and black pepper to taste

Instructions:
1. Quinoa should be combined with water or vegetable broth in a medium-sized saucepan. After bringing to a boil, lower the heat to a simmer, cover, and cook the quinoa for 15 to 20 minutes, or until it is tender and fluffy. Allow it to cool after you have taken it off the fire.

2. Put the cooked quinoa, cherry tomatoes, cucumber, bell pepper, red onion, parsley, and mint leaves (if using) in a big mixing dish. Gently toss to mix.

3. To make the lemon vinaigrette, combine the extra virgin olive oil, lemon juice, Dijon mustard, minced garlic, honey or maple syrup (if desired), salt, and black pepper in a small bowl.

4. Cover the quinoa and vegetable combination with the lemon vinaigrette, tossing to coat everything evenly.

5. Taste and adjust the seasoning with salt and black pepper, if needed.

6. If using, sprinkle the crumbled feta cheese over the salad just before serving.

Nutritional Information (per serving):
- Calories: 240 kcal
- Carbohydrates: 28 g
- Protein: 6 g
- Fat: 12 g

- Fiber: 4 g
- Sodium: 180 mg

Stuffed Potatoes with Salsa & Beans

Ingredients:
- 4 medium-sized potatoes (such as russet or sweet potatoes)
- One can of 15 ounces rinsed and drained black beans
- 1 cup salsa (homemade or store-bought)
- 1 avocado, diced
- 1/4 cup chopped fresh cilantro
- 1/4 cup diced red onion
- 1 lime, cut into wedges
- Salt and black pepper to taste
- Optional toppings: Greek yogurt or sour cream, shredded cheese, hot sauce

Instructions:
1. Set oven temperature to 400°F, or 200°C. Use parchment paper to line a baking sheet.

2. Give the potatoes a good wash and give them a fork prick all over. After putting them on the baking sheet that has been prepared, bake them for 45 to 60 minutes, or until a fork inserted into the potatoes comes out soft.

3. Make the filling while the potatoes are baking. The black beans, salsa, sliced avocado, chopped cilantro, and diced red onion should all be combined in a medium-sized bowl. To taste, add salt and black pepper for seasoning. Mix thoroughly to blend.

4. After the potatoes are cooked, take them out of the oven and let them cool down a little before handling them.

5. Cut each potato in half lengthwise, taking care not to sever the potato completely. Mash the insides of each potato half with a fork.

6. Evenly distribute the bean and salsa mixture among the potato halves by spooning a fair amount over each one.

7. For an added flavor boost, squeeze a slice of lime over each stuffed potato half.

Nutritional Information
- Calories: 280 kcal
- Carbohydrates: 50 g
- Protein: 9 g
- Fat: 5 g
- Fiber: 11 g
- Sodium: 460 mg

CHAPTER 8: DINNER- FISH AND SEAFOOD

Moroccan Baked Tilapia

Prep Time: 15 minutes
Cook Time: 20 minutes
Servings: 4

Ingredients:
- 6 oz/170g each of 4 tilapia filets
- 2 tablespoons olive oil
- 2 cloves garlic, minced
- 1 teaspoon ground cumin
- 1 teaspoon paprika
- 1/2 teaspoon ground coriander
- 1/2 teaspoon ground cinnamon
- ¼ tablespoon of
 cayenne pepper - Salt and pepper to taste
- 1 lemon, sliced
- Fresh cilantro, chopped, for garnish (optional)

Instructions:
1. Set oven temperature to 400°F, or 200°C. Apply cooking spray or olive oil sparingly to a baking dish.

2. Combine the olive oil, minced garlic, paprika, ground cumin, ground coriander, ground cinnamon, cayenne pepper, salt, and pepper in a small bowl.

3. Put the tilapia filets into the baking dish that has been ready. Evenly coat both sides of each filet by brushing it with the spice mixture.

4. Place lemon slices over the filets of tilapia.

5. Bake for 15 to 20 minutes in a preheated oven, or until the tilapia is thoroughly cooked and flake readily with a fork.

6. When the tilapia is done, take it out of the oven and, if you'd like, top it with freshly cut cilantro.

7. Serve hot, accompanied by your choice of sides such as steamed vegetables or couscous.

Nutritional Information (per serving):
- Calories: 180 kcal
- Protein: 24g
- Carbohydrates: 3g
- Fat: 8g
- Saturated Fat: 1g
- Cholesterol: 60mg
- Sodium: 120mg
- Fiber: 1g
- Sugars: 0g

Ingredient Substitutions:
- Substitute tilapia with another mild white fish like cod or sole.

Salmon Rice Bowl

Prep Time: 15 minutes
Cook Time: 25 minutes
Servings: 4

For the Salmon:
- 1 lb (450g) salmon filets, skin on
- 2 tablespoons olive oil

- 2 cloves garlic, minced
- 1 teaspoon ground ginger
- 2 tablespoons low-sodium soy sauce
- 1 tablespoon honey or maple syrup
- 1 tablespoon rice vinegar
- Salt and pepper to taste
- Sesame seeds for garnish (optional)

For the Rice Bowl:
- 2 cups cooked brown rice
- Two cups of chopped mixed vegetables such as bell peppers, broccoli, and carrots
- 1 tablespoon olive oil
- 2 tablespoons low-sodium soy sauce
- 1 tablespoon rice vinegar
- 1 teaspoon sesame oil
- Salt and pepper to taste
- Sliced green onions for garnish (optional)

Instructions:
1. Set oven temperature to 400°F, or 200°C. Apply cooking spray or olive oil sparingly to a baking dish.

2. Combine the olive oil, minced garlic, paprika, ground cumin, ground coriander, ground cinnamon, cayenne pepper, salt, and pepper in a small bowl.

3. On the baking sheet that has been prepared, place the salmon filets skin-side down. Make sure the salmon is evenly coated after pouring the marinade over it. Give it ten minutes or so to marinate.

4. Bake the salmon for 12 to 15 minutes, or until it is cooked through and flakes readily with a fork, in the preheated oven. Take out of the oven and, if you'd like, top with sesame seeds.

5. In a big skillet set over medium heat, warm up the olive oil while the salmon bakes. When the vegetables are crisp-tender, add the mixed ones and sauté for 5 to 7 minutes.

6. Combine the sesame oil, rice vinegar, soy sauce, salt, and pepper in a small bowl. After pouring the sauce over the veggies, toss to ensure even coating. Simmer for a further two to three minutes.

7. To assemble the rice bowls, divide cooked brown rice among serving bowls. Top each bowl with sautéed vegetables and a portion of baked salmon.

8. Garnish with sliced green onions, if desired, and serve immediately.

Nutritional Information (per serving):
- Calories: 400 kcal
- Protein: 25g
- Carbohydrates: 30g
- Fat: 20g
- Saturated Fat: 3g
- Cholesterol: 60mg
- Sodium: 500mg
- Fiber: 4g
- Sugars: 6g

Ingredient Substitutions:
- Substitute brown rice with quinoa or cauliflower rice for a lower-carb option.
- Replace soy sauce with tamari or coconut aminos for a gluten-free alternative.

Parmesan-Crusted Halibut with Spicy Brussels Sprouts

Prep Time: 15 minutes
Cook Time: 20 minutes
Servings: 4

For the Parmesan-Crusted Halibut:
- 4 halibut filets (about 6 oz/170g each), skin removed

- 1/4 cup grated Parmesan cheese
- 2 tablespoons almond flour or breadcrumbs
- 1 teaspoon dried thyme
- 1/2 teaspoon garlic powder
- Salt and pepper to taste
- 1 tablespoon olive oil

For the Spicy Brussels Sprouts:
- 1 lb (450g) Brussels sprouts, trimmed and halved
- 2 tablespoons olive oil
- 1 teaspoon smoked paprika
- 1/2 teaspoon chili powder
- Salt and pepper to taste

Instructions:

1. . Set oven temperature to 400°F, or 200°C. Apply cooking spray or olive oil sparingly to a baking dish.

2. Combine the grated Parmesan cheese, almond flour or breadcrumbs, dried thyme, garlic powder, salt, and pepper in a small bowl.

3. Put the tilapia filets into the baking dish that has been ready. Evenly coat both sides of each filet by brushing it with the spice mixture.

4. Bake the halibut filets for 12 to 15 minutes, or until it is cooked through and flakes readily with a fork, in the preheated oven.

5. Make the spicy Brussels sprouts while the halibut is baking. Brussels sprouts should be well coated after being mixed with olive oil, smoked paprika, chili powder, salt, and pepper in a big bowl.

6. Arrange the seasoned Brussels sprouts in a single layer on a second parchment paper-lined baking sheet. Bake for 15 to 20 minutes, stirring occasionally, or until the sprouts are soft and caramelized.

7. Once the halibut and Brussels sprouts are done, remove them from the oven. Serve the Parmesan-crusted halibut alongside the spicy Brussels sprouts.

Nutritional Information (per serving):

- Calories: 320 kcal
- Protein: 30g
- Carbohydrates: 12g
- Fat: 17g
- Saturated Fat: 3g
- Cholesterol: 70mg
- Sodium: 260mg
- Fiber: 5g
- Sugars: 2g

Ingredient Substitutions:

- Replace halibut with another firm white fish like cod or sea bass.
- Substitute almond flour with coconut flour for a nut-free option.

Lemon Garlic Salmon Bites

Prep Time: 10 minutes
Cook Time: 15 minutes
Servings: 4

Ingredients:

- 1 lb (450g) salmon filets, skin removed, cut into bite-sized cubes
- 2 tablespoons olive oil
- 3 cloves garlic, minced
- 2 tablespoons fresh lemon juice
- 1 teaspoon lemon zest
- 1 teaspoon dried oregano
- Salt and pepper to taste
- Fresh parsley, chopped, for garnish (optional)

Instructions:

1. Turn the oven on to 375°F, or 190°C. A baking sheet can be lightly oiled with olive oil or lined with parchment paper.

2. Combine olive oil, minced garlic, lemon zest, juice, dried oregano, salt, and pepper in a small bowl.

3. Transfer the salmon cubes to a mixing bowl and cover them with the marinade made of lemon and garlic. To evenly coat the fish, toss gently.

4. Thread the salmon cubes, with a small gap between each piece, onto skewers or toothpicks.

5. Put the skewers on the prepared baking sheet and bake for 12 to 15 minutes, or until the salmon flakes easily with a fork, in a preheated oven.

6. Once done, remove the salmon bites from the oven and garnish with chopped fresh parsley, if desired.

Nutritional Information (per serving):
- Calories: 240 kcal
- Protein: 25g
- Carbohydrates: 2g
- Fat: 14g
- Saturated Fat: 2g
- Cholesterol: 70mg
- Sodium: 80mg
- Fiber: 0.5g
- Sugars: 0g

Ingredient Substitutions:
- For a dairy-free option, substitute olive oil for butter.

CHAPTER 9: DINNER-MEAT/POULTRY RECIPES

Pepper and Tomato Sirloin Steak

Prep Time: 15 minutes
Cook Time: 15 minutes
Servings: 4

Ingredients

- About 6 oz each of 4 sirloin steaks trimmed of excess fat
- Salt and black pepper, to taste
- 2 tablespoons olive oil
- 1 onion, thinly sliced
- 2 bell peppers sliced thinly
- 2 cloves garlic, minced
- One can of 14.5 oz drained diced tomatoes
- 1 teaspoon dried oregano
- 1 teaspoon paprika
- Fresh parsley, chopped, for garnish (optional)

Instructions

1. Give the sirloin steaks a liberal amount of salt and black pepper on both sides.

2. Heat the olive oil in a sizable skillet or grill pan over medium-high heat.

3. Add the seasoned sirloin steaks to the skillet and cook to the desired doneness, about 3–4 minutes each side for medium-rare. After taking the steaks out of the skillet, set them aside.

4. Add the bell peppers and onion, cut thinly, to the same skillet. Simmer for 3–4 minutes, or until tender.

5. Fill the skillet with the minced garlic, paprika, and dried oregano. Sauté for a further one to two minutes, or until aromatic.

6. Add the chopped tomatoes that have been drained, making sure to scrape away any browned remains from the skillet's bottom.

7. For five minutes, simmer the ingredients over medium-low heat to enable the flavors to mingle and the sauce to slightly thicken.

8. Put the cooked sirloin steaks back in the skillet and tuck them into the mixture of tomato and pepper. Over the steaks, spoon the sauce.

Nutritional Information (per serving)
- Calories: 350 kcal
- Protein: 40g
- Carbohydrates: 10g
  - Fiber: 3g
  - Sugars: 5g
- Fat: 15g
  - Saturated Fat: 4g
- Cholesterol: 100mg
- Sodium: 300mg

Lamb Leg with Fresh Herbs

Prep Time: 15 minutes
Cook Time: 1 hour 30 minutes
Servings: 6

Ingredients
- 1 leg of lamb (about 3-4 pounds), bone-in and trimmed of excess fat
- Salt and black pepper, to taste
- 2 tablespoons olive oil
- 4 cloves garlic, minced
- 2 tablespoons chopped fresh rosemary

- 2 tablespoons chopped fresh thyme
- 1 tablespoon chopped fresh mint
- Zest of 1 lemon
- Juice of 1 lemon
- One cup of low-sodium vegetable broth or chicken broth
- Fresh herbs for garnish (optional)

Instructions

1. Turn the oven on to 375°F, or 190°C.

2. Using paper towels, pat dry the lamb leg. On all sides, liberally season with salt and black pepper.

3. Combine the olive oil, lemon zest, juice, chopped fresh rosemary, thyme, mint, and minced garlic in a small bowl. Well combined to form a paste of herbs.

4. Using your fingertips, evenly coat the entire lamb leg with the herb mixture.

5. Transfer the spiced lamb leg to a baking dish or roasting pan. Fill the pan's bottom with the low-sodium chicken or veggie broth. Put foil over the pan.

6. Bake the lamb for one hour in a preheated oven. After that, take off the foil and roast for a further half hour or until the internal temperature reaches your desired level of doneness (145°F/63°C for medium-rare, 160°F/71°C for medium).

7. Once cooked to your liking, remove the lamb from the oven and let it rest for 10-15 minutes before slicing. This allows the juices to redistribute and the lamb to become more tender. If desired, Garnish with fresh herbs before serving.

Nutritional Information (per serving)
- Calories: 350 kcal
- Protein: 45g
- Carbohydrates: 2g
  - Fiber: 0g
  - Sugars: 0g

- Fat: 17g
  - Saturated Fat: 5g
- Cholesterol: 150mg
- Sodium: 200mg

Ingredient Substitutions
- Substitute lamb leg with boneless lamb shoulder for a more budget-friendly option.

Cherry Chicken Lettuce Wraps

Prep Time: 20 minutes
Cook Time: 15 minutes
Servings: 4

Ingredients
- 1 tablespoon olive oil
- 1 pound ground chicken
- 1 small onion, finely chopped
- 2 cloves garlic, minced
- 1 cup finely chopped and pitted cherry cherries
- 1/4 cup low-sodium soy sauce (or, a gluten-free alternative, tamari).
- 2 tablespoons rice vinegar
- One tablespoon honey or any other sugar
- 1 teaspoon grated ginger
- Salt and black pepper, to taste
- 1 head iceberg or butter lettuce, leaves separated

For Garnish (optional)
- Sliced green onions
- Chopped fresh cilantro
- Sesame seeds

Instructions

1. Heat the olive oil in a big skillet or wok over medium-high heat.

2. Add the ground chicken to the skillet and cook, breaking it up with a spoon, for 5 to 7 minutes, or until it is browned and cooked through.

3. Add the minced garlic and chopped onion and stir. Simmer the onion for two to three minutes, or until it is transparent and tender.

4. Fill the skillet with the chopped cherries, rice vinegar, low-sodium soy sauce, grated ginger, honey, or sugar substitute (if using), and salt and black pepper. Mix thoroughly to blend.

5. Lower the heat to medium-low and simmer the mixture for five to seven minutes, giving the sauce a chance to thicken a little and the flavors to combine.

6. To make lettuce wraps, spoon the cherry chicken mixture into each leaf individually.

7. Garnish the lettuce wraps with sliced green onions, chopped fresh cilantro, and sesame seeds if desired.

Nutritional Information
- Calories: 250 kcal
- Protein: 20g
- Carbohydrates: 15g
  - Fiber: 3g
  - Sugars: 10g
- Fat: 12g
  - Saturated Fat: 2.5g
- Cholesterol: 80mg
- Sodium: 450mg

Marinated Grilled Chicken with Zucchini

Prep Time: 15 minutes
Marinating Time: 1 hour
Cook Time: 15 minutes
Servings: 4

Ingredients

- About 4 oz each of 4 boneless chicken breasts
- 2 medium zucchini, sliced into rounds
- Salt and black pepper, to taste

For the Marinade

- 1/4 cup low-sodium soy sauce (or, a gluten-free alternative, tamari).
- 2 tablespoons olive oil
- 2 tablespoons lemon juice
- 2 cloves garlic, minced
- 1 teaspoon dried oregano
- 1 teaspoon dried basil
- 1/2 teaspoon paprika

Instructions

1. Combine together the low-sodium soy sauce, olive oil, lemon juice, minced garlic, dried oregano, dried basil, and paprika in a small bowl.

2. Transfer the chicken breasts to a shallow dish or a plastic bag that can be sealed. Make sure the chicken is evenly coated after pouring the marinade over it. To allow the flavors to develop, cover or seal the dish/bag and refrigerate for at least one hour, but preferably overnight.

3. Turn the heat up to medium-high on your grill.

4. Shake off any excess marinade before removing the chicken breasts. Throw away any leftover marinade. To taste, add a pinch of salt and black pepper to the chicken. After the grill has heated up, put the chicken on it and cook it for 6 to 8 minutes on each side, or until it is cooked through and no longer has pink in the middle. A temperature of 165°F (74°C) should be reached internally.

5. Add the sliced zucchini rounds to the grill while the chicken cooks. Cook for 2-3 minutes per side, or until tender and lightly charred.

6. Remove the grilled chicken and zucchini from the grill. Let the chicken rest for a few minutes before slicing it. Serve the marinated grilled chicken with zucchini hot, alongside your favorite side dishes or a fresh salad.

Nutritional Information (per serving)
- Calories: 250 kcal
- Protein: 30g
- Carbohydrates: 6g
  - Fiber: 2g
  - Sugars: 3g
- Fat: 10g
  - Saturated Fat: 2g
- Cholesterol: 80mg
- Sodium: 400mg

Baked Chicken with Onions and Leek

Prep Time: 15 minutes
Cook Time: 45 minutes
Servings: 4

Ingredients
- 4 oz each of 4 boneless skinless chicken breasts
- Salt and black pepper, to taste
- 1 tablespoon olive oil
- 1 onion, thinly sliced
- 1 leek, trimmed and thinly sliced
- 2 cloves garlic, minced
- 1 teaspoon dried thyme
- 1/2 cup of low-sodium chicken broth
- Juice of 1 lemon

- Chopped fresh parsley, for garnish (optional)

Instructions

1. Turn the oven on to 375°F, or 190°C.

2. Use salt and black pepper to season the chicken breasts on both sides.

3. Heat the olive oil in a sizable oven-safe skillet over medium-high heat. When golden brown, add the chicken breasts and cook for 3–4 minutes on each side. Keep the chicken after taking it out of the skillet

4. Add the leek and onion, cut thinly, to the same skillet. Simmer for 3–4 minutes, or until tender. Cook for an additional one to two minutes, or until aromatic, after adding the minced garlic and dried thyme.

5. Add the lemon juice and low-sodium chicken broth to the skillet, scraping to remove any brown pieces from the pan's bottom.

6. Nestle the seared chicken breasts back into the onion and leek mixture in the skillet. After transferring the skillet to the oven, warm it and bake for 25 to 30 minutes, or until the chicken reaches an internal temperature of 165°F (74°C), or cooked through.

7. Take it out of the oven and give it some time to rest. If desired, top the hot baked chicken with onions and leek with freshly cut parsley.

Nutritional Information (per serving)
- Calories: 250 kcal
- Protein: 30g
- Carbohydrates: 8g
  - Fiber: 2g
  - Sugars: 3g
- Fat: 10g
  - Saturated Fat: 2g
- Cholesterol: 80mg
- Sodium: 150mg

Beef Barley Skillet

Prep Time: 15 minutes
Cook Time: 40 minutes
Servings: 4

Ingredients
- 1 tablespoon olive oil
- One pound lean ground beef, should be at least 90% lean
- 1 onion, diced
- 2 cloves garlic, minced
- 1 carrot, diced
- 1 celery stalk, diced
- 1 cup pearl barley, rinsed
- 2 cups low-sodium beef broth
- 1 teaspoon dried thyme
- Salt and black pepper, to taste
- 2 cups fresh spinach leaves

Instructions
1. Heat the olive oil in a big skillet over medium heat.

2. Add the ground beef to the skillet and cook, breaking it up with a spoon, for 5 to 7 minutes, or until it is browned and cooked through.

3. Add the minced garlic and chopped onion and stir. Simmer the onion for two to three minutes, or until it is transparent and tender.

4. Fill the skillet with the rinsed pearl barley, diced carrot, and diced celery. Mix thoroughly with the mixture of beef.

5. Cover the mixture with the low-sodium beef broth and garnish with the dried thyme. To taste, add salt and black pepper for seasoning. Mix thoroughly.

6. Simmer the mixture for a while. Reduce the heat to low and place a lid on the skillet. Simmer for thirty to thirty-five minutes, or until, the barley is tender and most of the liquid is absorbed.

7. Once the barley is tender, stir in the fresh spinach leaves. Cook the spinach for a further two to three minutes, or until it wilts

Nutritional Information (per serving)
- Calories: 380 kcal
- Protein: 25g
- Carbohydrates: 40g
  - Fiber: 8g
  - Sugars: 3g
- Fat: 13g
  - Saturated Fat: 4g
- Cholesterol: 55mg
- Sodium: 320mg

Cheesy Asparagus Chicken Cutlets

Prep Time: 15 minutes
Cook Time: 20 minutes
Servings: 4

Ingredients
- Four skinless, boneless chicken breasts, each weighing about 4 oz.
- One bunch of asparagus, trimmed and chopped into 2-inch pieces; one tablespoon olive oil
- One cup of mozzarella cheese, shredded;
- One tablespoon of unsalted butter
- One tablespoon of all-purpose flour (for a whole grain option, use whole wheat flour).
- 1/4 cup grated Parmesan cheese
- 1/4 teaspoon garlic powder

- 1 cup low-sodium chicken broth
- To taste, add salt and black pepper.

Instructions

1. Set the oven temperature to 375°F, or 190°C.

2. Sandwich the chicken breasts between two pieces of plastic wrap or parchment paper. Gently pound the chicken to an equal thickness of about 1/2 inch with a meat mallet or rolling pin. Sprinkle salt and pepper on both sides of the chicken breasts.

3. Heat the oil in a big oven-safe skillet. Add the chicken breasts and cook for 3-4 minutes on each side until golden brown. Remove the chicken from the skillet and set aside.

4. In the same skillet, add the bits of asparagus. Cook until just beginning to soften, 3 to 4 minutes. Take out and place aside from the skillet.

5. Melt the butter in the skillet over medium heat. After one minute, whisk in the flour and cook. To avoid lumps, add the chicken broth gradually while whisking continuously. Add the garlic powder and Parmesan cheese and stir. Add pepper and salt for seasoning. Simmer the sauce for 2 to 3 minutes, or until it slightly thickens.

6. Nestle the asparagus and chicken breasts back into the sauce by adding them back to the skillet. Top with a scattering of mozzarella cheese shreds.

7. Place the pan in the preheated oven and bake for ten to twelve minutes, or until the chicken is cooked through and the cheese is bubbling and melted (165°F or 74°C on the inside).

Nutritional Information (per serving)
- Calories: 320 kcal
- Protein: 33g
- Carbohydrates: 6g
  - Fiber: 2g
  - Sugars: 2g

- Fat: 18g
  - Saturated Fat: 7g
- Cholesterol: 100mg
- Sodium: 520mg

CHAPTER 10: DINNER- SOUP RECIPES

Lentil and Vegetable Soup

Prep Time: 15 minutes
Cook Time: 30 minutes
Servings: 6

Ingredients
- 1 tablespoon olive oil
- 1 onion, finely chopped
- 2 cloves garlic, minced
- 2 carrots, peeled and diced
- 2 celery stalks, diced
- 1 bell pepper (any color), diced
- One cup of rinsed dried green or brown lentils
- Six cups of low-sodium vegetable broth
- One can of 14.5 ounces diced tomatoes, with juices
- 1 teaspoon dried thyme
- 1 teaspoon dried oregano
- Salt and pepper, to taste
- Fresh parsley, chopped (for garnish)

Instructions
1. Heat the olive oil in a big pot or Dutch oven over medium heat. Add chopped onion and cook until softened, about 3 to 4 minutes. Cook the minced garlic for a further one to two minutes.

2. Add the rinsed lentils and diced carrots, celery, and bell pepper. Simmer for 3–4 minutes, or until the veggies are starting to get tender.

3. Stir in diced tomatoes (with liquids) and low-sodium vegetable broth. Add oregano and dry thyme for seasoning. The lentils should be soft after 25 to 30 minutes of simmering the mixture.

4. After tasting the soup, taste again and add more salt and pepper if necessary. Pour the Filling Lentil and Vegetable Soup into individual bowls. Add freshly cut parsley as a garnish.

Nutritional Information (per serving)
- Calories: 220
- Total Fat: 3g
  - Saturated Fat: 0.5g
- Cholesterol: 0mg
- Sodium: 380mg
- Total Carbohydrates: 40g
  - Dietary Fiber: 12g
  - Sugars: 8g
- Protein: 12g

Apple Chicken Stew

Prep Time: 15 minutes
Cook Time: 30 minutes
Servings: 6

Ingredients
- 1 tablespoon olive oil
- 1 onion, finely chopped
- 2 cloves garlic, minced
- 2 carrots, diced
- 2 celery stalks, diced
- 2 medium apples, diced
- One pound of boneless, skinless chicken breast, diced
- Four cups of low-sodium chicken broth

- 1 teaspoon dried thyme
- 1/2 teaspoon ground cinnamon
- Salt and pepper, to taste
- Fresh parsley, chopped (for garnish)

Instructions

1. Heat the olive oil in a big pot or Dutch oven over medium heat. Add chopped onion and cook until softened, about 3 to 4 minutes. Stir in the minced garlic, celery, and cubed carrots. Cook the veggies for a further two to three minutes, or until they are soft.

2. Add the diced apples and chicken breast. Allow the chicken to brown slightly by cooking it for 5 to 7 minutes.

3. Add chicken broth with reduced sodium. Add ground cinnamon and dried thyme for seasoning. Once the chicken is cooked through and the flavors have blended, bring the mixture to a simmer and cook for 15 to 20 minutes.

4. After tasting the apple chicken stew, taste it again and add more salt and pepper if necessary. Spoon stew mixture into bowls. Add freshly cut parsley as a garnish.

Nutritional Information (per serving)

- Calories: 250
- Total Fat: 7g
  - Saturated Fat: 1g
- Cholesterol: 60mg
- Sodium: 380mg
- Total Carbohydrates: 20g
  - Dietary Fiber: 4g
  - Sugars: 10g
- Protein: 25g

Tips

- For added richness, consider finishing the stew with a splash of low-fat milk or unsweetened almond milk.

- Serve this Apple Chicken Stew with a side of whole-grain bread or a crisp green salad for a complete meal.

Tortilla Soup

Prep Time; 15 minutes
Cook Time: 30
Servings: 4

Ingredients
- One tablespoon of olive oil
- One finely chopped onion;
- Two minced garlic cloves; one diced bell pepper (any color)
- One finely chopped jalapeño pepper (optional, for heat)
- One 14.5-ounce can of diced tomatoes with juice
- 1/2 teaspoon smoked paprika
- 1 teaspoon ground cumin
- 4 cups low-sodium chicken broth
- One-half teaspoon of chili powder
- One cup chopped or shredded cooked chicken breast
- One cup of fresh, frozen, or canned corn kernels
- One cup of rinsed and drained black beans
- Season to taste with salt and pepper - Finely slice fresh cilantro (for garnish)
- Chips or tortilla strips baked in the oven (for serving)

Instructions
1. Heat the olive oil in a big pot or Dutch oven over medium heat. Add chopped onion and cook until softened, about 3 to 4 minutes. Add the diced bell pepper, minced garlic, and jalapeño pepper (if using). Cook until aromatic, about 2 to 3 minutes more.

2. Add the low-sodium chicken broth and chopped tomatoes with their juices. Add chili powder, smoked paprika, and ground cumin for seasoning. To let the flavors combine, bring the mixture to a simmer and cook for ten to fifteen minutes.

3. Include the black beans, corn kernels, and cooked chicken breast in the saucepan, either shredded or diced. Simmer until thoroughly cooked, 5 to 7 minutes more.

4. After tasting the soup, taste again and add more salt and pepper if necessary. Spoon Tortilla Soup into individual dishes. Add a garnish of chopped fresh cilantro. Serve hot with baked tortilla strips or tortilla chips on the side.

Nutritional Information (per serving
- Calories: 280
- Total Fat: 7g
  - Saturated Fat: 1g
- Cholesterol: 30mg
- Sodium: 380mg
- Total Carbohydrates: 35g
  - Dietary Fiber: 8g
  - Sugars: 6g
- Protein: 20g

Ingredient Substitutions
- **Chicken Breast**: Substitute with cooked turkey breast or tofu for a vegetarian option.
- **Corn**: Use fresh, canned, or frozen corn kernels depending on availability.

Corn Chowder with Bacon

Prep Time: 15 minutes
Cook Time: 30minutes
Servings: 6

Ingredients
- 4 slices lean bacon, chopped
- 1 tablespoon olive oil
- 1 onion, finely chopped

- 2 cloves garlic, minced
- 2 carrots, peeled and diced
- 2 celery stalks, diced
- 4 cups fresh or frozen corn kernels
- 2 medium potatoes, peeled and diced
- 4 cups low sodium chicken broth
- One cup of unsweetened almond milk
- 1/4 cup of all purpose flour
- Salt and pepper, to taste
- Fresh chives, chopped (for garnish)

Instructions

1. Cook chopped bacon over medium heat in a large pot or Dutch oven until crisp. Using a slotted spoon, remove bacon and place on a dish covered with paper towels. Put aside.

2. If necessary, add olive oil to the same saucepan. Add chopped onion and cook until softened, about 3 to 4 minutes. Stir in the minced garlic, celery, and cubed carrots. Cook the veggies for a further two to three minutes, or until they are soft.

3. Add the diced potatoes and corn kernels, either fresh or frozen. Simmer for five to seven minutes to let the flavors combine.

4. Combine all-purpose flour and low-fat milk (or unsweetened almond milk) in another bowl and whisk until smooth. Stir the mixture continuously as you pour it into the pot.

5. Add low-sodium chicken broth gradually, stirring to blend. Bring the blend to a simmer and cook for 15-20 minutes, or until the potatoes are tender and the soup has thickened.

6. Season the Corn Chowder with Bacon with salt and pepper, to taste. Ladle the soup into bowls. Garnish with chopped fresh chives and reserved crispy bacon.

Nutritional Information (per serving)

- Calories: 280

- Total Fat: 8g
  - Saturated Fat: 2g
- Cholesterol: 15mg
- Sodium: 380mg
- Total Carbohydrates: 45g
  - Dietary Fiber: 6g
  - Sugars: 8g
- Protein: 10g

Ingredient Substitutions
- **Bacon**: For a vegetarian option, eliminate or replace with turkey bacon
- **Low-Fat Milk:** Use unsweetened almond milk or soy milk for a dairy-free option.

CHAPTER 11: DINNER- BEAN, RICE AND PASTA RECIPES

Creamy Brown Rice Risotto

Prep Time: 10 minutes
Cook Time: 40 minutes
Servings: 4

Ingredients:
- 1 cup brown rice
- Four cups of low-sodium vegetable broth
- 1 tablespoon olive oil
- 1 onion, finely chopped
- 2 cloves garlic, minced
- 8 ounces mushrooms, sliced
- 1/2 cup dry white wine (optional)
- 1/4 cup grated Parmesan cheese
- Salt and black pepper to taste
- Chopped fresh parsley, for garnish

Instructions:
1. The low-sodium vegetable broth should be simmered over medium heat in a medium saucepan. To keep the soup heated, turn the heat down to low.

2. Heat the olive oil in a different, sizable skillet or pot over medium heat. Add the finely chopped onion and simmer for approximately five minutes, or until transparent. Stirring constantly, cook for a further minute after adding the minced garlic.

3. When the mushrooms are golden brown and soft, add the sliced ones to the skillet and simmer for 8 to 10 minutes.

4. Add the brown rice and stir continuously for two to three minutes, or until the rice is lightly browned.

5. Add the dry white wine, if using, and stir until the rice absorbs it.

6. One ladleful at a time, add the warm vegetable broth to the skillet, stirring frequently and letting each addition absorb before adding more. Continue this process until the rice is cooked through and has reached a creamy consistency, about 30-35 minutes.

7. Once the rice is cooked, stir in the grated Parmesan cheese until melted and well combined. Season with salt and black pepper

8. Garnish with freshly cut parsley and serve hot

Nutritional Information (per serving):
- Calories: 240
- Total Fat: 6g
- Saturated Fat: 1.5g
- Cholesterol: 5mg
- Sodium: 380mg
- Total Carbohydrates: 35g
- Dietary Fiber: 3g
- Sugars: 3g
- Protein: 7g

Ingredient Substitutions:
- For a dairy-free option, omit the Parmesan cheese or substitute it with nutritional yeast for a cheesy flavor.
- Customize the risotto by adding additional vegetables such as spinach, peas, or roasted butternut squash according to personal preference and dietary needs.
- If dry white wine is not preferred, you can omit it or replace it with low-sodium vegetable broth.

Creamy Shrimp and Avocado Pasta

Prep Time: 15 minutes
Cook Time: 15 minutes
Servings: 4

Ingredients:
- 8 ounces whole-wheat spaghetti or pasta of choice
- 1 tablespoon olive oil
- 1 pound medium shrimp, peeled and deveined
- 2 cloves garlic, minced
- 1/4 teaspoon red pepper flakes (optional)
- 1 ripe avocado, pitted and diced
- 1/4 cup plain Greek yogurt
- 1/4 cup low-fat milk
- 2 tablespoons freshly squeezed lemon juice
- Salt and black pepper to taste
- Chopped fresh parsley, for garnish

Instructions:

1. First things first, let's get that whole-wheat spaghetti or your choice of noodles bubbling away just like the box says, until they're perfectly al dente. Once they're done, give them a good drain and pop them to the side for later.

2. Heat the olive oil in a big skillet over medium heat. Add the red pepper flakes (if using) and minced garlic, and sauté for one minute, or until fragrant.

3. Once the shrimp are pink and opaque, add them to the skillet and cook for two to three minutes on each side. Set the shrimp aside after taking it out of the skillet

4. Place the chopped avocado, plain Greek yogurt, low-fat milk, and freshly squeezed lemon juice in a blender or food processor. Blend till creamy and smooth. To taste, add salt and black pepper for seasoning.

5. Transfer the cooked pasta back to the skillet and cover it with the rich avocado sauce. Toss to distribute the sauce evenly over the pasta.

6. Add the cooked shrimp to the skillet with the pasta and sauce. Mix everything together gently until well cooked.

7. Serve hot garnished with chopped fresh parsley.

Nutritional Information (per serving):
- Calories: 380
- Total Fat: 12g
- Saturated Fat: 2g
- Cholesterol: 150mg
- Sodium: 280mg
- Total Carbohydrates: 42g
- Dietary Fiber: 8g
- Sugars: 2g
- Protein: 30g

Ingredient Substitutions:
- For a dairy-free option, use dairy-free yogurt or coconut cream instead of Greek yogurt and low-fat milk.

Caribbean Tofu with Black Beans and Rice

Prep Time: 15 minutes
Marinating Time: 30 minutes
Cook Time: 30 minutes
Servings: 4

For the Tofu Marinade:
- 1/4 cup orange juice
- 2 tablespoons low-sodium soy sauce
- 1 tablespoon olive oil

- 2 cloves garlic, minced
- 1 teaspoon ground cumin
- 1 teaspoon chili powder
- 1/2 teaspoon smoked paprika
- Salt and black pepper to taste
- 14 ounces firm tofu, pressed and cubed

For the Rice:
- 1 cup brown rice
- 2 cups water
- 1 tablespoon olive oil
- 1 onion, diced
- 1 bell pepper (any color), diced
- 1 can (15 ounces) black beans, drained and rinsed
- 1 teaspoon ground cumin
- 1 teaspoon dried thyme
- Salt and black pepper to taste
- Chopped fresh cilantro, for garnish

Instructions:
1. To make the marinade, combine the orange juice, low-sodium soy sauce, olive oil, minced garlic, ground cumin, chili powder, smoked paprika, salt, and black pepper in a shallow dish. Add the cubed tofu to the marinade, making sure it coats it well. Cover and refrigerate for at least half an hour to allow the flavors to mingle.

2. In a medium saucepan, combine the brown rice and water. Bring to a boil over high heat; lower the heat to low, cover, and simmer for 20 to 25 minutes, or until the rice is soft and the water is absorbed. Remove from heat and let sit, covered, for five minutes. Fluff the rice with a fork.

3. In a large skillet over medium heat, warm up olive oil while the rice cooks. Add the diced onion and bell pepper to the skillet and cook for 5-7 minutes, or until softened.

4. In a large skillet over medium heat, warm the olive oil while the rice cooks. Simmer the chopped onion and bell pepper in the skillet for five to seven minutes, or until they are tender.

4. Combine the marinated tofu with the onion and bell pepper in a skillet, along with any leftover marinade. Cook, stirring periodically, for 8 to 10 minutes, or until the tofu is crispy and golden brown on the edges.

5. Add the ground cumin, dried thyme, black pepper, salt, and rinsed and drained black beans. Cook until well cooked for another 3-4 minutes.

6. Serve hot, garnished with chopped fresh cilantro.

Nutritional Information (per serving):
- Calories: 380
- Total Fat: 12g
- Saturated Fat: 2g
- Cholesterol: 0mg
- Sodium: 480mg
- Total Carbohydrates: 50g
- Dietary Fiber: 8g
- Sugars: 3g
- Protein: 20g

Ingredient Substitutions:
- For a gluten-free option, ensure that the soy sauce used in the marinade is gluten-free.

CHAPTER 12: DINNER- VEGETARIAN RECIPES

Buttermilk Fried Tofu with Smoky Collard Greens

For the Buttermilk Fried Tofu:
- One block (14–16 ounces) of extra-firm tofu that has been drained and pressed
- One cup of plant-based buttermilk
- One tablespoon of hot sauce
- One cup whole wheat flour, or any other type of flour
- One tsp of paprika
- One-half teaspoon powdered garlic
- Half a teaspoon of powdered onion
- Salt and black pepper to taste
 - Use vegetable oil for frying

For the Collard Greens with Smoke:
- One bunch of collard greens, with the stems cut off and the leaves thinly sliced;
- One tablespoon olive oil
- Two minced garlic cloves
- One-half tsp smoked paprika
- 1/4 teaspoon (optional) red pepper flakes
- One cup veggie broth
- To taste, add salt and black pepper

Instructions:
1. To begin, prepare the tofu. Depending on your preference, slice or cube the pressed tofu.

2. Combine the spicy sauce and buttermilk in a small bowl. Make sure the tofu slices or cubes are completely covered by placing them in the buttermilk marinade. To get the most flavor, let them marinade for at least 30 minutes or up to overnight in the refrigerator.

3. Combine the whole wheat flour, paprika, onion, garlic, and black pepper powders in a different shallow dish. Toss to blend well.

4. In a skillet or frying pan, heat the vegetable oil over medium-high heat.

5. Working in batches if needed to prevent packing the pan too full, carefully drop the coated tofu pieces into the heated oil. Fry until crispy and golden brown, 3–4 minutes per side. To drain any extra oil, move the fried tofu to a platter covered with paper towels.

7. Make the smoky collard greens while the tofu is frying. Heat the olive oil in a big skillet or pot over medium heat. Add the red pepper flakes (if using), smoked paprika, and minced garlic. Simmer for one to two minutes, or until aromatic.

8. Include the cut collard greens in the skillet and toss to coat with the spiced oil. After adding the vegetable broth, boil the mixture.

9. Cook the collard greens in the skillet with a cover on for 15-20 minutes, stirring occasionally, or until they are tender and wilted. Season with salt and black pepper to taste. Serve and Enjoy!

Nutritional Information (per serving):
- Calories: 350 kcal
- Carbohydrates: 26 g
- Protein: 18 g
- Fat: 20 g
- Fiber: 6 g
- Sodium: 540 mg

Kale & Avocado Salad with Blueberries & Edamame

Ingredients:
- 4 cups thinly sliced kale with the stems off
- 1 chopped ripe avocado
- 1 cup rinsed and drained blueberries
- 1/4 cup of toasted almond slices (optional)
- 1 cup of cooked and cooled shelled edamame
- Two teaspoons of optionally shredded feta cheese

Dijon-Lemon Vinaigrette:
- Two tablespoons of fresh lemon juice
- 1/4 cup extra virgin olive oil
- One teaspoon Dijon mustard
- One chopped clove of garlic
- One teaspoon (optional) of honey or maple syrup
- To taste, add salt and black pepper.

Instructions:
1. Layer the sliced kale, diced avocado, blueberries, cooked edamame, and sliced almonds (if using) in a large mixing bowl.

2. Make the lemon Dijon vinaigrette in a small bowl by whisking together the extra virgin olive oil, fresh lemon juice, Dijon mustard, minced garlic, honey or maple syrup (if using), salt, and black pepper.

3. Pour the vinaigrette over the kale and avocado mixture, tossing gently to coat everything equally.

4. Before serving, sprinkle the crumbled feta cheese on top of the salad. Serve as a refreshing and nutritious meal or side dish.

Nutritional Information (per serving):
- Calories: 280 kcal
- Carbohydrates: 20 g
- Protein: 9 g
- Fat: 20 g
- Fiber: 8 g
- Sodium: 110 mg

Spinach Alfredo Lasagna

Ingredients:
- Nine whole wheat or gluten-free lasagna noodles, if preferred
- Ten ounces of thawed and drained frozen chopped spinach
- One tablespoon of olive oil
- Two chopped garlic cloves
- Two cups of homemade or store-bought low-fat Alfredo sauce
- 1/2 cup grated Parmesan cheese
- One cup of low-fat cottage or ricotta cheese
- 1/2 teaspoon dried basil
- 1/2 teaspoon dried oregano
- Salt and black pepper to taste
- One cup of shredded mozzarella cheese

Instructions:
1. Begin by warming the oven to 375°F (190°C) and lightly coating a 9x13-inch baking dish with either cooking spray or a brush of olive oil.

1. Prepare the lasagna noodles as per the instructions on the package until they reach an al dente texture. Once cooked, drain them and place them aside.

2. In a sizable skillet, warm some olive oil over a medium flame. Introduce the minced garlic and allow it to sauté for 1-2 minutes, until it emits a pleasant aroma.

3. Incorporate the defrosted and well-drained chopped spinach into the skillet. Let it cook for 3-4 minutes, stirring now and then, until the spinach is thoroughly warmed and any surplus liquid has been removed. Take the skillet off the heat and put it aside.

4. In a separate bowl, blend together the low-fat Alfredo sauce, low-fat cottage cheese or ricotta, grated Parmesan, dried basil, dried oregano, salt, and pepper. Stir the mixture until it is uniformly combined.

5. To construct the lasagna, spread a modest amount of the Alfredo sauce mixture across the base of the greased baking dish.

6. Lay down three lasagna noodles atop the sauce, slightly overlapping them to ensure the dish's bottom is completely covered.

7. Over the noodles, distribute half of the spinach mixture, followed by another layer of the Alfredo sauce mixture.

8. Continue layering with another three noodles, the rest of the spinach mixture, and an additional portion of Alfredo sauce.

9. Finish by placing the final three noodles on top, and cover them with the remaining Alfredo sauce mixture.

10. Evenly scatter the shredded mozzarella cheese over the lasagna's surface.

11. Seal the dish with aluminum foil and bake it in the oven, now at the set temperature, for 30 minutes.

12. Afterward, remove the foil and continue to bake for an extra 10-15 minutes, or until the cheese on top turns a bubbly golden brown.

13. Once baked, allow the Spinach Alfredo Lasagna to rest for a short while before cutting and serving.

Nutritional Information (per serving):

- Calories: 320 kcal
- Carbohydrates: 30 g
- Protein: 18 g
- Fat: 14 g
- Fiber: 3 g
- Sodium: 600 mg

CONCLUSION

Adopting a diabetic-friendly lifestyle is a proactive and empowering approach to managing diabetes and promoting overall health. By incorporating balanced nutrition, mindful eating practices, regular physical activity, and other healthy habits, individuals can optimize their well-being and reduce the risk of complications associated with diabetes.

It's important to remember that managing diabetes is a journey that requires dedication, patience, and ongoing education. Each small step towards healthier eating and lifestyle choices can make a significant difference in blood sugar control and overall quality of life. As a professional dietitian, I encourage you to continue exploring diabetic-friendly recipes, experimenting with nutritious ingredients, and embracing a variety of flavors and culinary techniques.

I want to express my gratitude to you for taking the initiative to learn more about diabetic-friendly nutrition and seeking ways to improve your health. Your commitment to making informed food choices and prioritizing your well-being is commendable and will undoubtedly have a positive impact on your health outcomes.

Remember, you are not alone on this journey. Connect with healthcare professionals, support groups, and resources available in your community to receive guidance, encouragement, and personalized advice tailored to your needs. Stay proactive in managing your diabetes by monitoring your blood sugar levels regularly, attending medical appointments, and staying informed about new developments in diabetes care.

Lastly, embrace the journey towards a healthier lifestyle with optimism and resilience. Celebrate your successes, learn from challenges, and stay motivated to prioritize your health and well-being. By making sustainable changes and maintaining a positive mindset, you are taking proactive steps towards living your best life with diabetes.

Thank you once again for your commitment to health and wellness. Together, let's continue to embrace a diabetic-friendly lifestyle and inspire others to make positive changes for a healthier future. Wishing you success and good health on your journey ahead!

<u>I Have A Request</u>

Dear Readers,

I hope you've been enjoying the delicious and healthful journey with my book, "Super Easy Diabetic Diet Cookbook After 50." I've poured my heart and expertise into creating a resource that makes managing diabetes simpler and more enjoyable for those over the age of 50.

Your feedback means the world to me! If you've had a chance to try out some of the recipes, I would be incredibly grateful if you could take a moment to share your thoughts. Your reviews not only help others who might be considering the book but also provide me with invaluable insights into how I can continue to serve you better.

Writing a review is easy and doesn't take long. You can share what you loved, your favorite recipes, or how this cookbook has made a difference in your daily routine. Every word you write is appreciated and helps to spread the word about living a healthier life with diabetes.

Please leave your review in English on the platform where you purchased the book or on any book review sites. Thank you for your support, and I look forward to reading your experiences and success stories!

Warm regards,
[Kimberly Mullins]

To stay updated on my latest releases, events, and behind-the-scenes insights, please visit my Author Central page at [https://www.amazon.com/author/mullinskimberly]. Discover more about my passion for creating delectable recipes, hosting memorable gatherings, and nurturing a love for the culinary arts. Thank you for your support, and may your culinary journey continue to be filled with joy and delicious discoveries!

SPECIAL BONUS

BONUS 1 & 2

"60 DAY MEAL PLAN + GROCERY SHOPPING LIST"

BONUS 3 & 4

"Diabetes Foot Care Tips"

BONUS 5

"Emergency Snack pack ideas & Diabetes Desserts"